D0728360

ORTHOREXIA

Praise for Renee McGregor's *Orthorexia*

"Renee's book provides a truly excellent description of orthorexia and how the search for health, if taken to excess, may lead psychological or even physical harm. Her approach is clear, nutritionally sound, and full of practical, sensible advice. I highly recommend it for anyone struggling to find the balance between healthy lifestyle and excessive restriction." – Dr Steven Bratman MD

"Essential reading for anyone who is concerned that their 'healthy' lifestyle is going too far... Renee McGregor brings expertise and empathy to this important subject. This book is accessible, authoritative and packed with first-rate practical advice." – Emma Woolf, *An Apple a Day*

"This book is timely and important. I am sure that it will be an invaluable resource – a lifeline for the many people affected by this poorly understood condition. But more than that, I hope that it will serve as a much needed wake up call, shining bright light upon the often damaging rhetoric of the wellness industry. Perhaps this is the intelligent and informed study that will inspire a new generation of wellness gurus to fully consider the consequences of the messages they spread."
– Anthony Warner, *The Angry Chef*

ORTHOREXIA

WHEN HEALTHY EATING GOES BAD

RENEE
McGREGOR RD

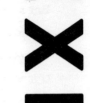

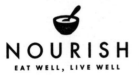

NOURISH
EAT WELL, LIVE WELL

Orthorexia: When Healthy Eating Goes Bad
Renee McGregor

This edition published in the UK and USA 2017 by
Watkins, an imprint of Watkins Media Limited
19 Cecil Court
London WC2N 4EZ

enquiries@nourishbooks.com

Publisher: Jo Lal
Managing Editor: Kate Fox
Project Editor: Judy Barratt
Production: Uzma Taj

10 9 8 7 6 5 4 3 2 1

Typeset by seagulls.net
Printed and bound by CPI Group (UK) Ltd, Croydon, CR0 4YY

A CIP record for this book is available from the British Library

ISBN: 978-1-84899-334-1

nourishbooks.com

CONTENTS

FOREWORD BY BEE WILSON

. . . .

Have there ever been such complicated times in which to eat? To walk through a modern city is to be bombarded with food *options* of one kind and another. There is a pulse of low-level anxiety around what we put in our mouths and what it will do to our bodies, with much talk of certain things being "good" (avocado, say) and even more talk of others being "bad" (sugar). Nor are we entirely wrong to look with suspicion on the modern food supply. Never before have so many people been sickened not by under-nutrition but over-nutrition, with galloping rates of Type 2 diabetes and other diet-related diseases across the globe. In our world "food" is everywhere, and yet has become something that we can no longer automatically count on to nourish us and keep us strong. No wonder that many of us have become confused and unhappy about the whole question of what to eat. It's tempting to believe that there is some set of perfect food rules out there that could make all our dilemmas go away.

Complicated times such as these are a gift to gurus promising easy solutions. But these solutions turn out to be less easy than they first seem. Nor are they real answers, but dangerous ideas that create a raft of fresh problems. If modern diets are lacking in vegetables then perhaps, suggest these gurus, the answer is a diet that consists of *nothing but* vegetables? Social media is full of wellness prophets promising us ultimate health – plus glowing skin! – if only we can relinquish all carbohydrates and sugars and live on such ingredients as coconut oil, kale and spiralized vegetables. Our brains are assaulted with endless mixed messages about food. It ought to be such a source of uncomplicated delight, a universal human pleasure, so it is sad that for so many people, eating itself has become instead something to feel perpetually guilty about and scared of. Anyone trying to develop a balanced relationship with food has to find their own path between the extremes.

Fear of food is a perfectly understandable response to the food environment we now inhabit, particularly for anyone who is going through other life stresses. But it's also a deeply damaging and disordered mindset to get into, as Renee McGregor explains so calmly and knowledgably in this timely book. Orthorexia nervosa – a disorder in which individuals fixate on "correct" eating to the point where they are severely restricting their intake – may not be as well known as anorexia nervosa, but it can be both physically and mentally debilitating for those suffering from it. What makes orthorexia even harder to diagnose and treat is that to many in the outside world, orthorexic forms of behaviour look normal or even praise-worthy. For the past couple of years, the bestseller lists for food in Britain have been dominated by "clean eating" books (although many of the authors themselves have now disowned the phrase). It has become almost mainstream to suggest that the way to achieve good health is to cut out entire categories of food, ranging from bread to sugar to gluten to all carbohydrates.

What does "clean eating" even mean? The definitions vary depending on who's talking and what they are selling. For some Instagram gurus, "clean eating" is always vegan and "plant based", whereas to others, it includes certain kinds of meat. But the basic idea is that there is somehow a perfectly pure way of eating which will keep you safe from harm and perhaps even guarantee you longevity. Most clean eating "experts" advise basing your diet on the freshest, most organic vegetables, the most cold-pressed and extra-virgin oils. This sounds good – after all, most of us could stand to eat a few more vegetables and a bit less sugar – but as Nigella Lawson has wisely commented, "clean eating" is based on a fatally flawed view of both food and of life. As Lawson wrote in 2016, "Food is not dirty, the pleasures of the flesh are essential to life. We cannot control life by controlling what we eat."

I spoke to a young woman in her early twenties who said that the experience of having a meal out with friends had been ruined by our culture's love affair with "clean eating". Every time she tried to order something from the menu, one or other of her friends would pass judgement on the choice, and suggest that she might opt for something "better": something vegan, something lacking in wheat or dairy, something raw, something with sweet potatoes instead of ordinary potatoes. Even though she disagreed with these little interventions, and continued to order the pasta that she really wanted, she found that her enjoyment of dinner was marred. Unlike anorexia, which is generally suffered in a state of secrecy, orthorexic behaviour, as Renee McGregor notes in the book, is often flaunted in public.

For the sake of both mental health and good food, we need to fight with every bone in our bodies the idea that there is such a thing as a "perfect" ingredient or indeed a perfect way of eating. Enjoying a varied diet is not something we should feel guilty about, but a vital and life-enhancing part of being human. "Clean eating" – so far from being healthy – is a kind of spurious anti-food because it encourages you to ignore your senses and to be scared of nourishment.

This book is a marvellously useful and wise guide in that fight, whether you are someone who feels themselves slipping into orthorexia or whether you are concerned about a friend or family member who is displaying signs of worrying food restrictions. No one is better qualified to write about this subject than Renee McGregor, whose work as a dietitian has involved working with many eating disorder sufferers, as well as with Olympic athletes. Hers is a voice of authority and practical wisdom, an antidote to so much of the nonsense that is spouted in the name of "nutrition". If you want to know why "non-refined" sugars are no better for you than the refined white kind or why needlessly restricting gluten is a bad idea or why many nut milks are little better than expensive water, this is the book for you. I've never read a clearer explanation of why carbohydrates, so far from being some kind of a dietary demon, are actually a useful source of energy. But the thing I like best of all about the book is its tone of compassion. So

INTRODUCTION

. . . .

"Food! Glorious food!"

Isn't this what eating should be about? Personally, I think the lyrics to this song, written for the musical adaptation of Charles Dickens's *Oliver Twist*, are very poignant – through them, we can see how our attitude toward food has changed since the time when orphans in 18th-century workhouses dreamt of being able to fill their bellies with "cold jelly and custard", rather than measly gruel.

During Dickens's time, there was a great deal of poverty. Glorious food was the province of the wealthy upper classes, a symbol of success. To have abundant dietary choice represented robust and healthy stature. Fast forward to the present day and we seem to be more concerned with which foods we should avoid; improved social status sometimes appears to be related to how much we can pare down our diet. In effect, at times we seem to have gone from "Look at how brilliant I am with this feast of plenty" to "Look at how brilliant I am – I can live on a lettuce leaf a day".

When did this all change? Why has food become such a minefield? Should we be cutting back on nutrients? Should we believe all the scaremongering? How have we got to the stage where so many people in the developed world have lost their unadulterated enjoyment of glorious food?

Food has always played a central role in bringing people together; from cavemen gathering around their fires to roast the catch of the week, to families coming together for a special occasion, or even just a weekly get-together with friends on a Sunday. Food not only provides physical, but also emotional nourishment.

An increase in ethnic diversity has brought our cuisine new flavours, spices, colours, ingredients and combinations, providing us with an ever-evolving menu of culinary possibilities. Food is – or at least it should be – exciting, inventive and creative. Why then has it become such a bitter dish for so many people?

As the culinary adventure has gathered pace, so too has our understanding of how the human body works, and – among myriad other things about that wonderful human machine – nutrition. We know more about not only what food the body needs for good health, but also why and how it needs it than we have ever known before. And yet there is still so much confusion – is this a case where improved knowledge has rather muddied the nutritional waters? When we were eating according to what was available and in line with our instincts (that is, according to what our body was telling us we needed), were things just simpler and so, perhaps, healthier?

It's easy to hark back and think that things were better "then". The truth is that probably they weren't. Knowledge *is* power – we just have to use that power in the right way. My belief is that when a little nutritional knowledge is misunderstood or misinterpreted, or nutritional luck is misrepresented as nutritional fact, we have a problem. And that's what I think happens with orthorexia.

This disease, not yet officially recognised as an eating disorder, but with all the attributes of one, is characterised by the quest to purify the self through dietary rules and regimes; simply, it is defined as an obsession with healthy eating.

3

Eating disorders are not a new phenomenon and yet they continue to be so misunderstood. They are often associated with girlish teenage fads – in fact, they affect both genders and all ages. They are often thought of as superficial or whimsical, but in fact they are a form of deeply rooted self-harm – punishment is in the form of food restriction, purging, or in the case of orthorexia nutritional deprivation to the point of malnourishment. (It is startling, I think, to know that anorexia nervosa has the highest rate of mortality of all mental illnesses.) They are thought to be primarily about physical image, but in fact many eating disorders are the symptom of a need to numb pain and turmoil that has nothing to do with physicality and everything to do with what's going on inside a sufferer's head. Fundamentally, all eating disorders – orthorexia included – are multi-factorial mental illnesses.

This book provides me with an opportunity to use my nutritional knowledge and vast experience working with both athletes and those with eating disorders to help untangle some of the crossed wires relating to food and nutrition, in the context of orthorexia nervosa. Primarily, it is a book to highlight this growing illness, to help people to recognise it perhaps in themselves or others, but also in the growing, increasingly scary potential for it in a modern world that makes information and misinformation so readily accessible, and where social media provides us with unsubstantiated miracle cures at every click.

This book is not intended primarily as a self-help book (overcoming orthorexia requires individualised, professional help from both mental health experts and dietitians, so a book can go only so far), although inevitably it has elements of self-help about it. Its main purpose is to educate, re-educate and raise awareness.

In the first chapter we'll look at what orthorexia is, how it earned its name, what its causes and symptoms might be, and its place among the other, better-known eating disorders. In Chapter 2, we'll look at some of the most common dietary fads and regimes that I have seen so often provide the rule-book for sufferers of orthorexia. We'll look at the science behind what those diets are actually doing to the body – for better or worse – and consider how each one can cause a slide into an unhealthy, malnourished way of life that is dangerously repackaged as the pursuit of purity. In Chapter 3, I'll share my own expertise on what healthy eating actually means in terms of what goes onto your plate (spoiler alert: it's not glamorous, but it *is* good for you) and how to use the orthorexic mindset to reset the dietary rules for a truly healthy way of life with the aim of starting on the path to true wellness and genuine freedom from disordered eating. And, finally, in Chapter 4, I'll round off with advice for how to find professional help if you think you or someone you know may be suffering from orthorexia, and what hopes I have for the future when it comes to further opening up the debate, undertaking more research and highlighting this debilitating and serious condition of modern times.

In short, this book is an explanation of how healthy eating goes bad, and what (I hope) we can do about it.

CHAPTER 1

DEFINING ORTHOREXIA

Ask a roomful of 100 people what you mean by the word "orthorexia" and most of them will look back at you perplexed, perhaps even confused. Certainly, when I've told people about the most recent book I'm writing, I've been met mostly with baffled expressions. That's okay: it is, after all, a relatively new term and describes what is fundamentally a relatively modern problem.

So, what is orthorexia? What does it mean and where does the word come from?

In 1996 Dr. Steven Bratman, a medical doctor in San Francisco, USA, coined the term orthorexia nervosa to describe patients whom he had identified as having become obsessed with healthy eating. *Ortho* comes from the Greek prefix meaning right or correct; and "orexia" from the Greek *orexis* meaning appetite or desire. So, whereas anorexia means "without appetite" (*an* meaning without), orthorexia means "correct appetite". The suffix *nervosa* means "obsession". So, orthorexia nervosa describes obsession with "correct" eating. While Dr. Bratman never intended his new term to be used as a diagnosis, over time he found that it did indeed legitimately identify an eating problem.

Fast forward a decade and while the term orthorexia is still not officially recognised as an eating disorder in the *Diagnostic and Statistical Manual of Mental Disorders* (the *DSM-5*; see box opposite), it has many of the characteristics that we associate with one. Those who suffer from illnesses such as anorexia or bulimia nervosa obsess about calorie intake, weight, and body image. This obsession, though, is an outlet – a manifestation of a sufferer's need to transfer, control and overcome his or her underlying anxiety about and disharmony in the sense of self. In other words, these eating disorders are first and foremost mental illnesses, not physical ones.

The table on the following pages identifies the similarities and differences between orthorexia and the more well-documented eating disorders, anorexia and bulimia. It helps to show how orthorexia sits in the spectrum of illness. Furthermore, each of these conditions often goes hand in hand with obsessive–

compulsive disorder (OCD) tendencies (see pages 10–12).

WHAT IS THE *DSM-5*?

Having taken more than a decade to put together, the *DSM-5* is the combined expertise of hundreds of international experts in all fields of mental health. Their incredible, comprehensive and rigorous work has resulted in a volume that defines and classifies mental disorders in order to improve diagnoses, treatment and research.

At the time of writing, the volume was last updated in 2013 by the American Psychiatric Association and serves as the universal authority for psychiatric diagnosis. It has significant practical importance as it provides practitioners with treatment recommendations.

While both anorexia nervosa and bulimia nervosa appear in the directory, orthorexia nervosa as yet does not. However, with further updates sure to happen in the future, there are positive signs that orthorexia will become a fully recognized and clinically categorized illness.

	Anorexia Nervosa	
What is it?	• Obsessive fear of weight gain and conviction that the sufferer is overweight. • Restricting food intake to reduce total calories consumed. • May also have odd rituals around food.	
Body image	• Convinced that they are fat, even when body shape and weight is below normal ranges acceptable for height and age. • Distorted body image.	
Physical symptoms	• Refusal to maintain bodyweight at a minimally normal weight for age and height – for diagnostic purposes, this means weight loss to the extent that a person weighs 85% less than you'd expect for their age and height. • As a result, sufferers may also display low blood pressure, fainting, loss of menstruation in women, hair loss, fatigue.	

Bulimia Nervosa	Orthorexia Nervosa
• Recurrent episodes of binge eating – consuming a large amount of food in a short period of time – followed by purging by vomiting, laxitives, medication or fasting. • Binge eating and purging occur at least twice a week on average.	• Obsessive adherence to an increasingly restrictive, "clean" diet. • Restricting food intake based on a perception of the "purity" of ingredients. • May also include excessive exercising.
• Although weight loss may be less pronounced than in anorexia, sufferer similarly cannot assess body shape or weight objectively. • Distorted body image.	• Weight loss is often less pronounced than in anorexia, sufferer similarly cannot assess body shape or weight objectively. • Distorted body image. • Focus on skin quality ("glow") and tone as well as body size.
• Body mass usually normal or overweight for age and height. • As a result of purging, sufferers may also have mouth ulcers and dental issues, fluctuating weight, halitosis, dehydration, fatigue.	• Body mass usually normal for age and height. • Restrictions in "impure" foods mean that certain food groups are removed – carbohydrate, gluten or dairy – without medical reason. • Dietary restriction may result in nutritional deficiencies, which can manifest in loss of menstruation, fatigue, headaches, anaemia. digestive issues, halitosis in certain cases.

	Anorexia Nervosa	
Emotional symptoms	• Depression, anxiety, obsessive–compulsive behaviours, intense fear of gaining weight or situations where eating is required. • Body dysmorphia – inability to see body shape and weight as it is.	

The diagram opposite demonstrates how anorexia, orthorexia and obsessive–compulsive disorder (OCD), while existing as conditions in their own right, also have huge overlaps in terms of their symptoms and characteristics. They are especially similar when it comes to the key personality traits and behaviours that seem to predispose individuals to each of the conditions. There's more on orthorexia and OCD on pages 35–41.

While an orthorexic might not look in the mirror and see a distorted body image that he or she feels compelled to rectify through controlling food intake, he or she will obsess about healthy eating as a method

DEFINING ORTHOREXIA

Bulimia Nervosa	Orthorexia Nervosa
• Depression, anxiety, self-loathing, guilt. • Feelings of lack of control during eating – the sufferer doesn't feel able to stop.	• Depression, anxiety, self-loathing, guilt, intense fear of eating types of food that are not 'pure'. • Obsession with dietary rule-following – going to great lengths (and often expense) to consume food deemed 'healthy'. • May experience body dysmorphia – inability to see body shape and weight as it is. • May have an unhealthy obsession with exercise.

ORTHOREXIA

• Focus on food quality
• Unrealistic food benefits
• Desire to maximize health
• Feelings of superiority

• Inability to reason
• Guilt over breaking food rules
• Pursuit of idealized self-image
• Lack of self-awareness

• Rituals relating to food preparation
• Obsession with food contamination

• Perfectionism
• Intrusive thoughts
• Anxiety
• Working memory and focus problems
• Inability to read situations or empathize

ANOREXIA

• Focus on food quantity
• Body dysmorphia
• Preoccupation with becoming obese
• Obsessive exercising to lose weight

• Secretive behaviour
• Low mood or depression

OCD

• Obsessive behaviours relate to any aspect of life
• Self-awareness
• Behaviour inconsistent with self-image

of trying to achieve a positive sense of self through a process and perception of being pure. In some cases, an illness is the trigger – "If I cut out sugar from my diet, I will recover from..." or "If I no longer eat carbohydrate, I'll stop suffering from..." One way or another, a sense of improving well-being leads to the obsessive pursuit of a "pure" or "clean" diet.

Over time, the symptoms of orthorexia have expanded not just to include what a sufferer is prepared to eat, but also how a sufferer approaches exercise (see box below) and well-being in general. Therefore, we could say that we know now that orthorexia is obsessiveness not just about pure eating, but about pure living, too.

THE ROLE OF EXERCISE

I don't want to lay all responsibility for the increase in orthorexia at the door of attitudes to food (or food fads – see pages 58–114). We are also bombarded with information – some good, some not-so-good – about how important it is that we exercise in order to maintain good health. When you're looking for ways to become "pure", exercise can become as much of an obsession as food.

Governments in the UK and US give the following broad guidelines on activity levels for healthy adults. Of course, if you do more than these guidelines, the benefits to your health are improved, as long as your exercise routine remains within healthy parameters.

- At least 2½ hours a week of moderate aerobic activity, during which you work at a pace that allows you to have a conversation but makes you slightly out of breath; as well as including some bodyweight strength exercises, such as press-ups, squats, sit-ups, or classes providing, say, yoga or pilates, at least twice a week.

Or

- 1¼ hours of vigorous aerobic exercise a week during which you are working as hard as you can and can manage only a few words between breaths. In addition, you should include some bodyweight or strength work using weights (free or machine) at least twice a week.

Or

- A mixture of the above aerobic workouts for at least 2½ hours a week with strength sessions at least twice a week.

These are good, healthy parameters for exercise in the average adult. However, when exercise starts to control the way in which a person behaves (perhaps he or she misses important appointments or social events in order to fit in an exercise session; or he or she has exercise-related pain but ignores it and pushes on regardless), something is going wrong. When there's no moderation or flexibility, and no self-compassion when the body screams for change – when routine becomes regime – there is a lack of good judgement and of good health. That, then, indicates illness manifesting as obsessive behaviour.

A WORLD OF MISINFORMATION

Of course, all this begs the question: where does the belief that "pure" or "clean" eating or living, according to skewed principles, leads to optimal health and well-being come from?

Thinking just about nutrition for now, every day
it seems we are bombarded with new messages
about what foods are good for us. On the one hand,
we might read newspaper articles reporting on a
new study that has discovered that certain foods
or cooking styles "cause" cancer. On the other, we
might come across government health initiatives
aimed at combatting obesity, diabetes and other
illnesses that are becoming more common in
developed communities. We all know that sugar, salt
and saturated fat consumed to excess are bad for
our health. The good thing about any government
initiatives and research articles is that – on the whole
– press and public announcements are made after
rigorous longitudinal, scientific studies. (Not always –
but mostly.) Put simply, more or less we can trust that
they are grounded in some scientific fact.

However, there's a third – and in my view a more
dangerous – world of information that's emerging.
One of misinformation.

Over the last five years, we've seen a massive increase
in numbers of people who have shared their incredible,
wonderful, heart-warming success stories for good
health through social media, websites and blogs.

Whether it's been a gluten-free diet that's allegedly "fixed" migraines or a sugar-free diet that's "cured" ME, there are claims a-plenty for the miracle-working of specific dietary rules for specific ailments. I love it that people are looking for naturopathic ways in which to improve their health and well-being, but I don't advocate claims of miracle cures.

"What's the problem?" I hear you say. "If it's healthy and it worked for him or her…?" The short answer is that there's no problem – as long as healthy eating doesn't become obsessive to the point that the rules of those diets begin to control a way of life. But, that's not always the case.

First, anyone who is ill or run down or overcome with low self-esteem is vulnerable. Have you ever felt so poorly – say, with a sore throat, or a cold, or a stomach bug – that you would try any old wives' tale to try to feel better? In most cases, and for most illnesses, that's completely harmless. You'll feel better anyway once your immune system kicks in and you may or may not put it down to that one particular piece of ancient wisdom you decided to try during your most desperate moments. It doesn't really matter – you're better and that's what counts.

But, what if that vulnerability meant that you completely bought into unsubstantiated, unscientific claims about the ability of a particular nutritional approach to cure you of something more serious? Or, to fill a deep yearning to feel good about yourself or an all-consuming need to take control of your life? Whether it's a chronic physical illness, or something intangible – a psychological illness, like the illnesses that trigger anorexia or bulimia – "getting better" is a far more involved, complex process that can take not just months, but many years, and perhaps even a lifetime to overcome. It might involve medical treatment, or psychological therapy. When the immune system isn't providing the natural path to getting better, there's no particular end in sight for pursuing the unfounded claims of modern-day nutritional "gurus". For the orthorexic mind, this means endless, obsessive pursuit of a rainbow's end that might not produce the pot of gold. It's exhausting and depleting and unhealthy.

The net result of a bombardment of information and misinformation is a jumble of confusion and contradiction – and yet more vulnerability for those who are already vulnerable.

Many clients come to my clinic completely unaware that their strict, controlled methods of eating and exercising may be, at best, having no effect on their physical well-being at all or, at worst, doing more harm than good. On the contrary, they sit proudly in front of me and announce that they have gone gluten-free or are using agave in place of refined sugar, or have completed a half-marathon three times this week. My response is always the same: why do you think that's healthy? I ask: are you sure you're doing the best for your body? I'm often met with utter deflation (and sometimes I'm met with anger) when I have to say that rigorous rule-following, even in the name of better health, for someone who is fundamentally physically healthy already, isn't actually healthy at all. In fact, it might itself be the cause of illness.

CASE STUDY

THE HARMFUL SEARCH FOR PERFECTION

A young woman in her 20s came to see me. She had landed a high-profile city job that demonstrated how brilliant she was in her profession. As the demands of the job increased, so did her need to be perfect in every sense. Worried about the effects of alcohol on her body, she started to avoid going out with work colleagues; she removed sugar, then bread and finally all carbohydrates from her diet. She ate no dairy. Her diet was basically a small piece of chicken or fish and a plate of spiralized vegetables twice a day every day. She became isolated, emotionally unstable and exhausted, but still she could not allow herself to deviate from her chosen nutritional path.

She contacted me because she had had a well-woman check at work that showed that her levels of cholesterol were higher than they should be for her age and weight. She wanted to know what else she could do to bring this level down – after all, as far as she was concerned she had already removed all the damaging foods from her diet.

Her story perfectly highlights the interrelatedness of our body systems. While on the surface of it she was eating a very healthy, lean diet, it was completely without balance. The side-effect was that her endocrine system had stopped functioning properly. I discovered that she was no longer making sufficient amounts of oestrogen, the "female" hormone that not only plays such a crucial role in a woman's fertility, but also metabolizes fat and protects against cardiovascular disease because it regulates the production of cholesterol. With her levels of oestrogen so low, my client's body had no trigger to mitigate its production of cholesterol, so her cholesterol just kept going up. She found this a very difficult concept to understand – after all, in her mind her very "healthy" diet could not be causing her harm. Once she got it, though, she could start a road to recovery.

OBJECTIVITY AND FEAR

This brings us to an important point. A person who has orthorexia cannot objectively view what it means to have a healthy lifestyle. In orthorexia, eating and exercise are not relaxed, enjoyable pastimes, but regimes with strict rules. For someone with orthorexia, the thought of breaking the rules invokes feelings of fear – a sense that something catastrophic will happen if any single rule is broken at any time, even just as a one-off. In reality, the fear is irrational, but it *feels* completely logical.

It's the obsessive way in which a person with orthorexia follows the rules that is the problem – not necessarily the rules themselves. After all, eating more fruits and vegetables, less sugar, fewer refined foods, less saturated fat and so on are all good dietary principles. But, when all objectivity is lost and fear has taken hold, reducing saturated fat can easily, over time, become eliminating all fat; cutting back on sugar can become eliminating all carbohydrate (see page 69 for why); increasing vegetables can become eating only vegetables. In other words, obsessiveness is cumulative and ongoing – what could be healthy, over time with further pushing on the boundaries, becomes harmful and even dangerous.

REDEFINING HEALTHY EATING

In an ideal world I would have all literature relating to "Healthy Eating Guidelines" redefined as "Healthy Attitudes to Eating". Whenever I talk about healthy eating, I try to make clear that by that I mean unrestrained and uncomplicated eating. I don't mean bingeing – I mean eating a sensible, balanced diet according to the body's nutritional needs (which means eating from all the major food groups, as well as stocking up on important nutrients; see pages 52–6) *most* of the time. To me "unrestrained eating" means not feeling guilty or fearful if occasionally something nutritionally imperfect – perhaps something indulgent like a chocolate bar or a bowl of ice cream – passes your lips. A healthy attitude is about having a fact-based understanding of nutrition, and feeling confident enough to relax the guidelines every now and then and know that, on balance and considered over weeks and months rather than hours or days, you have a healthy diet.

Last year I went away with some friends to the Dolomites in Italy for a week. We chose to have pastries for breakfast every morning. Now, I don't usually eat pastries for breakfast, nor do I usually eat them every day, but I was on holiday and I wanted to enjoy the experience of breaking from the norm. Did anything awful happen to me? No. On the contrary, it was good to have a change; and I felt more relaxed and restored when I came home. I didn't suddenly become addicted to pastries for breakfast – I went back to my healthier choices without a second thought. In my view, this is healthy eating. And it's this we need to promote, rather than diets with strict and restrictive rules that may not always be beneficial to health and well-being. Did I just tell you that you could have that biscuit with your cup of tea? I certainly did! Just try not to eat the whole packet, every day...

WHAT CAUSES ORTHOREXIA?

Orthorexia is about obsessive self-improvement, rather than necessarily doggedly trying to reach a perfect weight, as in the more well-known eating disorders such as anorexia and bulimia. The aim is to improve the self through improved quality in diet and lifestyle, rather than to reduce, restrict or burn calories. That said, there are clear commonalities in the triggers for obsessive, extreme behaviours between all three eating disorders. We might say that these are the fundamental underlying factors – "causes" is probably too limiting a word – of orthorexia (and of anorexia and bulimia).

Feelings of being out of control

We can't control how anyone else looks or feels. Nor can we control everything that happens to us over the course of a day, week, year or life. Dissatisfaction with life and the self, and feeling impotent to put it right or to have influence over it, means that a vulnerable person may turn to food intake as something he or she can control to try to find order in everything else that feels out of kilter or unmanageable. We see this in small children all the time – think of the toddler who copes day in, day out with being told what to do and how to behave, probably even what to wear. Then, it comes to teatime and he or she flatly refuses to eat a carrot, or a piece of broccoli, or a piece of chicken. Why? Because when so much feels out of control, what we put into our bodies is something over which we *can* have the final word. Mouth clamped shut, what can we do?

It's the feelings of being out of control that lead to obsessive, predictable patterns of behaviour – whether that manifests as a strict diet or a particular order for completing a certain task. It's not surprising that those with an eating disorder also often show other obsessive–compulsive tendencies, too (see diagram, page 13).

Low self-esteem

Purging the body in order to rid it of feelings of inadequacy or incompleteness manifests in anorexics as abstinence, in bulimics as regurgitation, and in orthorexics as eating purely according to the strict rules of a chosen diet. Of course, nothing about low self-esteem is as simple as all that. Feelings of not being good enough often have deep roots, embedded in years of perceived failure, or perhaps trauma or anxiety and stress. Nonetheless, a set of food rules, closely followed at all times, provides a sense of success and fulfilment – "If I can adopt these rules and live by them at all times, I must be good enough because I have succeeded."

CASE STUDY

THE ROLE OF SELF-ESTEEM

I worked with a teenager a few years ago who suffered from acne. It made her feel very self-conscious and her self-esteem was very low. She started researching on the Internet for ways to reduce the spots on her skin. The first thing she did as a result of her research was to remove all foods high in sugar and fat, including sweets and chocolates. When this had very little effect on her acne (there is, in fact, no evidence that sugar causes acne), she next took out dairy, then gluten, then all meat and animal-derived products. That is, she became vegan. In general I have no issue with veganism, except that in this case, the girl also insisted on being sugar-free and low-fat, and she refused to use soya products to provide protein as she had read that these would be harmful to her body in other ways.

She was probably the most extreme case of orthorexia I have come across. No matter what advice I gave her and no matter how scientific my reasons for that advice, she chose to believe what she was reading on the Internet. Once she could do no more with her diet, she started looking for other ways to help herself. She joined a gym, which soon also became an obsession – she often attended two sessions a day and would become very anxious if school work got in the way. She constantly refused social invitations as these would interfere with not only her eating rules, but also her exercise rules.

She came to me because while she thought she was doing everything right, she wasn't seeing the adaptations or results she was looking for in her body. When I explained to her that while she thought she was following an optimal diet, in reality it was insufficient in energy, protein or fat to support her training. Although her weight was fairly stable and within normal parameters for her age, weight and height, her menstruation had stopped. This was a huge indicator that her body was not functioning optimally. However, in the end it was getting a boyfriend that convinced her to change her pattern of behaviour. The change in priorities was enough to convince her to gradually break the orthorexic mindset. Her self-esteem improved and she wanted to be able to socialize with her boyfriend. She agreed to limit her exercise sessions and increase her intake of carbohydrate. Her periods came back and her acne reduced (as a result of medication, rather than dietary changes), but it took several months before she could understand that no one food or food group had been able to "cure" her, and instead she needed to achieve balance – physical, psychological, hormonal and also social.

A need to be perfect

One study, published in *Eating and Weight Disorders (EWD) Journal* in April 2016, investigated the causes of orthorexia. The researchers asked 220 individuals to complete a questionnaire investigating attitudes to perfectionism, body image, relationships and self-esteem. The results found that, as well as a previous history of eating disorder, there were higher orthorexic tendencies in those showing higher scores in dissatisfaction with body image and a need for perfection. Of course, this makes sense – the (skewed) logic goes that through the perfect and precise following of rules comes a perfect person.

Lack of self-compassion

I have found that one of the most striking and recurring themes that comes up during my work with individuals who have disordered-eating issues, such as orthorexia, is lack of self-compassion, the inability to be kind to the self. When we are healthy, we know that there is no such thing as perfect – there isn't the perfect journey, the perfect meal, the perfect cup of coffee, let alone the perfect body. We forgive life for its anomalies and imperfections and we even appreciate and welcome them as the flecks of colour in every otherwise ordinary day. For a person with orthorexia, however, as we've seen there is a need to be perfect. When perfect doesn't come, instead of a quick shrug of the shoulders, there is guilt, remorse, self-loathing. Someone with orthorexia keeps pushing, even if the body screams to stop (in pain or hunger or because of some other physical need); there's a sense that we are not worthy of our own kindness, because we aren't yet good enough – perfect enough – to deserve it.

These triggers are by no means exhaustive. Just as every individual has different dietary needs, so every individual has different psychological pushes, pulls and touchpoints. I couldn't pretend to have covered them all, nor even to have discovered them all – but these are the triggers that I see so frequently in the clients who come to my clinic.

THE EXTERNAL TRIGGER: INFORMATION RED ALERT

In this chapter I have tried to define orthorexia in terms of its characteristics, its symptoms and its possible causes. There is one important external trigger that I have to mention because I think it is the one that – as outsiders, or as people who are worried about loved ones developing the illness – we can actually influence.

We know that among the triggers for eating disorders is the pursuit of perfection – in the way we look, feel and behave. Indeed, recent studies suggest that children as young as six years old are unhappy with their looks – with such pressure at such a young age, we can only imagine what that's doing to the statistics for eating disorders later on in life. So, where does the idealism for that come from? How is it perpetuated?

In the past the fashion industry, magazines and media images of models have all been blamed for the rise in our sense of dissatisfaction with ourselves. Statistics show that:

- 85 per cent of fashion/beauty magazine content has the effect of making readers feel imperfect and inadequate.

- 75 per cent of women feel guilty, ashamed and depressed after only 3 minutes of reading a fashion magazine.

- The majority of women who read fashion magazines are over 40 years old and yet typically only a mere third of the images represent this age-group – the other two-thirds are of women who are significantly younger.

Today, as well as the images we see in print, we have social media to contend with. The core social-media websites (Facebook, Snapchat, Instagram and Pinterest, among others) have collected more than 100,000,000 registered users. More than 60 per cent of 13–17-year-olds have at least one profile on social media, with many spending more than two hours a day on social networking sites. Although we don't yet have clear statistics mapping the demographics of orthorexia, my own research and experience tells me that this age-group is also significantly susceptible to the notion of obsessive clean eating, with many teenagers dressing up their restricted food choices as vegetarianism or veganism with ethical justifications (see also page 101). Furthermore, social media has made it all-too-easy and accessible to be inspired by skewed representations of success and "perfection". Sites make it easier than ever to follow – and even create – trends and fads. Images of beautifully prepared, "clean" food; toned and slender bodies; and even muscle-toning workouts are accessible at all times in glorious technicolour. We are constantly subjected to ways in which to scrutinize our bodies, lifestyles and health; our sense of self-worth is under relentless pressure.

We live in a wonderful age of information – the Internet gives us instant access to all sorts of knowledge that might have taken days to find only a matter of decades ago. However, the great and grave danger of such accessible information is that not all of the information we can access is necessarily well researched or well founded. It all comes back to the old adage: don't believe everything you read. We all love a good rags-to-riches or illness-to-health story; we are all searching for answers to the secrets of beauty, youth and longevity. So, when young, impressionable and vulnerable individuals see a blog, vlog or web page seeming to claim how "if you eat like me, you can be like me" (usually that's gorgeous, successful and in every way brilliant), it's no wonder that one click becomes a thousand clicks, and one follower soon becomes ten-thousand followers and suddenly what was a deeply personal and deeply individual story of well-being becomes something that provides rules that apparently apply to all. Think about this in scientific terms – one person's story of a nutritional change that has resulted in renewed health and a greater sense of well-being is a study conducted on a cohort of one. There are no scientific studies with only one research subject; to even propose such a thing would be laughable. What works for one person is highly unlikely to work for all.

I'm not saying that there is no value in the advice that social-media people have to offer; I'm just saying that when anyone can write anything and make a story out of it, beware. Being dairy-free, for example, isn't the answer to the world's health crisis. In most people, it is more likely to lead to low levels of calcium and healthy fats and the associated health problems (weakened bones, and hormonal imbalance among other things); it's just that in a few people, those who are genuinely lactose intolerant, it can provide a path to wellness.

Be sceptical: over the last few years there have been a number of high-profile bloggers who have admitted that the lifestyle and images they created on social media were in fact quite different from their reality. One blogger explained how she took a photo of her abs more than 100 times in order to get the right angle to demonstrate how toned they were. Another spoke about how she posted images of green juices that she claimed made her feel wonderful, but at the same time she failed to mention that she couldn't stand the taste of them. Another spoke about how he had to photoshop his prepared meal so that it looked appetizing in the photograph, but in reality it was so horrible to taste that as soon as he'd taken the photograph, he put the food in the bin.

As I said, don't believe everything you read.

THE SYMPTOMS OF ORTHOREXIA

For a person suffering from an eating disorder, it is virtually impossible to notice that something is wrong – decisions to limit, restrict or in another way control food intake, when explained, can seem perfectly rational and logical and in the case of orthorexia, even healthy. That's why it's so important that we are all aware of the signs and symptoms – so that even if we can't see the dangers in our own behaviour, we can notice them in those we love. The following are some of the common signs in the behaviour of those with orthorexic tendencies.

Citing undiagnosed food allergies as rationale for avoiding certain foods

Individuals struggling not just with orthorexia but with any eating disorder may use this as an excuse to limit or control what they eat. In some individuals there is a categorical belief that a particular food or food group causes illness. However, others present it as an excuse – a means of sidestepping questions about what he or she is choosing to eat and not eat. For example, if I told you I was gluten-intolerant, you would be far less likely to question why I refuse a bowl of pasta or avoid eating the bread roll with the soup you've served me. Fabricating an allergy or intolerance enables sufferers to persist with the rules of their eating disorder even when they are with other people.

ANYTHING BUT MODERATE

There is nothing moderate or rational about the diet of an orthorexic. Someone with orthorexia will go out of their way to avoid food groups and ingredients, and even processes involved in food production, often without any rigorous understanding of under what circumstances these food groups might be nutritionally unhealthy for us (and therefore also why in some cases the body might in fact need them for health). In orthorexia, there's a banned list that might include all or some of the following:

- Fat, sugar or salt
- Animal or dairy products
- Foods containing any artificial colours, flavours or preservatives
- Foods treated with pesticides or having undergone genetic modification

Showing signs of co-occurring disorders, such as obsessive–compulsive disorder (OCD)

As we've already seen, the need to take control over life is a key trigger for eating disorders. This can manifest in food choices and also in other ways. Individuals who have OCD and an eating disorder often have set rules relating to food preparation (the way in which vegetables are chopped, the order in which ingredients are added, or the precise weighing of ingredients, for example), as well as obsessive attention to cleaning routines and even constant checking to ensure that they've done what they think they've done (checking and rechecking that you've locked the door, or folded the washing, or turned off the oven, for example). The routines of the disorder evoke a sense of control and calm. Any deviation from those routines causes anxiety and stress.

Performing elaborate rituals relating to food

Commonly, individuals with eating disorders will demonstrate extreme behaviour relating to food storage and (as I mentioned above) preparation. In addition, an individual with an eating disorder may create delicious and elaborate meals for other people, without eating a morsel themselves. On the one hand, this is a means to show compassion toward others to fulfil a need to demonstrate kindness that the sufferer finds it impossible show to him- or herself. On the other hand, it also gives the sufferer a sense of self-worth; or a feeling of somehow being superior to all those who can't resist the food that's put in front of them and don't follow those strict rules.

Evident discomfort eating food cooked by someone else

Remember how needing to take control is a trigger for orthorexia? Well, this manifests frequently in obvious signs that a meal cooked by someone else is somehow unpalatable or inedible. You might find that a sufferer will push food around his or her plate; or he or she may have hovered awkwardly in the kitchen while you're preparing the meal, watching every move.

Turning down social invitations that involve eating
Whether it's the birthday cake at a family gathering, or a three-course meal at a dinner party, those who suffer from eating disorders will avoid at all costs social situations that might involve the need to eat outside of their rules.

Healthy individuals often associate going out for dinner with friends as a means of bringing a sense of fulfilment to life. But, what makes that occasion a happy one? Is it the food? Probably not – it's the interactivity, the sociability, the human connection and the feeling of being part of a pack, of belonging. The great irony is that sufferers of orthorexia remove themselves from social situations, especially those involving food, because it's much harder to follow the food rules when someone else is doing the cooking or when other people are watching or perhaps questioning. The resulting sense of isolation goes on to create a vicious circle of low self-esteem and feelings of lack of self-worth.

Expressing guilt about breaking rules –
and trying to put things right

Remember that orthorexia is all about rule-following, so if any rule is broken the sense of guilt in the sufferer can be overwhelming. As a result he or she may show a particularly manic episode of exercise or food restriction somehow to redress the balance, purge and purify. If a friend says to you, "I can't come for a coffee because I have to go for a run/am fasting that day because I really overindulged yesterday", beware.

SPOTTING THE SIGNS

If you are worried about yourself or a friend and believe that orthorexia may be a problem, here is a summary list of signs to look out for:

- Elimination of entire food groups in attempt for a "clean" or "perfect" diet
- Severe anxiety regarding how food is prepared
- Avoidance of social events involving food for fear of being unable to comply with diet
- Thinking critically of others who do not follow strict diets
- Spending extreme amounts of time and money on meal planning and food choices

- Feelings of guilt or shame when unable to adhere to diet standards
- Feeling fulfilled or virtuous from eating "healthily" while losing interest in other activities
- Fear that eating away from home will make it impossible to comply with diet
- Distancing the self from friends or family members who do not share similar views about food
- Avoiding eating food bought or prepared by others
- Worsening depression, mood swings or anxiety
- Needing to exercise daily in order to justify eating

Even if you identify only with one or two of these signs, it's worth raising the alarm – or at least logging the thought. Remember that orthorexia is a sliding-scale condition – it will worsen over time, so it's important to be aware of the warning signs.

PERPETUATING THE CLEAN-EATING MYTHS

The Internet provides a limitless resource of clean-eating rules for those suffering from orthorexia. Celebrity and self-promotional blogs reinforce every day how "worthy" it is to eat clean. So significant is their influence that even brands and advertising have begun to tap into our insecurities about certain foods, subliminally sending us messages about how "free-from" is altogether healthier.

For example, milk alternatives, such as almond, oat and hemp, are often marketed as a great source of dairy-free nutrition. In reality they are just expensive water. Shop-bought almond milk contains 0.1g of carbohydrate and 0.1g of protein per 100ml and is almost double the price for the same amount of cow's milk and yet considerably lower in nutritional value (100ml cow's milk contains about 4.8g carbohydrate and 3.2g protein, as well as calcium and other nutrients). Similarly, brands selling naturally gluten-free products, such as ice cream, rice and even body lotion, now advertise the fact that these products are gluten-free. Why? To increase sales. The more we hear or read these messages, the more we believe that the free-from options must be better for us – and the more we feed into the orthorexic mindset.

So what is the answer? How do we get change?

One way is to arm yourself with facts and build your emotional resilience so that you start making choices based on your own needs, not someone else's. The next chapter starts the process of arming you against the traps we so easily fall into when it comes to understanding how and why the human body needs certain foods.

CHAPTER 2

DIET AND NUTRITION – FINDING ORTHOREXIA'S FALSE GOLD

We've already identified that the term "healthy eating" is open to interpretation; and that what it means to one individual may be different to what it means to another. Even when we think we're clear what it means for us, how we interpret the term may evolve over time.

Let's take an example. Let's say you're someone who has a teaspoon of sugar in your tea. You probably already know that too much refined sugar isn't good for your health, but if this is your only vice and if you're drinking only one cup of tea a day, it's really not going to be a problem. If, though, you drink four or five, or even more, cups of tea a day, probably you need to make some small changes to minimise its effects (blood-sugar imbalance, hormone imbalance, weight gain and so on). If there are other hidden sugars in your diet (see below), the problems may be exacerbated.

The key point here is that it's not a problem that you take sugar in your tea, but it's the quantity of sugar in your overall diet that you need to change. A simple step toward a healthier lifestyle would be to either reduce the number of cups of tea you drink each day; or to stop adding sugar to them. For some individuals, this small adjustment may be as far as he or she needs to go to become "healthier". Others may decide to look deeper, thinking about other ways sugar creeps in and swapping a daily chocolate bar, for example, for a piece of fruit; or basing one meal a week on beans and pulses rather than meat and two vegetables. To use an old adage: there are lots of ways to skin a cat. There are all sorts of ways in which – once we understand what sugar is and where it comes from – we can make small adjustments to improve nutritional health.

The point is that "healthy eating" is never about deprivation or strict rules. It is about making sustainable, positive nutritional changes that improve individual health in the long term. Small changes are cumulative and effective, and far more sustainable. When those changes become obsessive or restrictive (when small changes become "big" changes that provide rules to live by), they stop being positive steps toward improved health and become an eating disorder justified by "false gold".

Because those suffering from orthorexia rarely set out to lose weight or change their appearance (remember it's about feeling and being pure, rather than necessarily being thin), it's very easy to hide this illness under the shroud of nutritional psychobabble. In my role as a clinical dietitian, this is one way I can help: I'm not qualified to treat the underlying psychology of the condition, but I can help to improve the effects with education about nutrition.

UNDERSTANDING THE FUNDAMENTALS

In order to understand what food we need to put into our body for optimum health, and why orthorexia leads to ill health, it is important to appreciate the fundamental processes that occur within the human body.

Food is fuel, and, of course, providing the body with energy is one the main reasons that we eat. However, that energy isn't simply to power the muscles – rather, it powers many different physiological processes, from the cardiovascular system (heart and circulation) and the endocrine system (hormones) to the neurological system (brain and nerves) and the digestive system –

and myriad processes in between. On top of that the nutrients in our food trigger, sustain and in other ways regulate hundreds of cellular biochemical processes and ensure optimum skeletal health, too.

THE BACKED-UP BODY

The body is resilient. Even when we remove whole food groups from our diet, our nutritional intake is poor and the body experiences stress, it has numerous back-up systems that enable it to continue to function, albeit sub-optimally. This is why it can be so difficult to identify an eating disorder such as orthorexia until the situation has become fairly extreme.

If we start to "control" our diet – either by restricting calorie intake or by following a diet that removes a certain food group – nutritional balance is lost. The body makes adjustments to preserve energy in order to maintain those systems that are necessary for life – those that control the brain, breathing and heart. While we may buy into the promise of glowing skin by swapping spaghetti for courgetti, what does this actually mean in terms of the chemistry of the body? What are the potential negative effects?

Over the following pages, I want to take a closer look at the importance of all the food groups in terms of overall good health. Then, I'll look at them in light of how restricting them in the diet, or even removing them altogether, can have important, unhealthy consequences that show that the pursuit of purity has been taken to the extreme. If you are worried about someone, or yourself, this is the toolkit you'll need to assess honestly diet claims you may be following, and to ask how healthy that diet really is in light of evidence-based nutritional science.

HOW YOUR BODY WORKS

Let's start with a quick biology lesson – we can't really understand the importance of nutrition unless we understand the basics of how the body is Nature's most intricate, interrelated and interdependent machine of all. The human body has 11 primary systems involved in optimal health. All of these need optimum nutrition in order to function properly and support each other.

The body's 11 main systems are:

- **The cardiovascular/circulatory system**, which is responsible for circulating blood around the body, delivering oxygen and nutrients to organs and cells, and removing waste products.

- **The digestive system**, which is necessary for the mechanical (chewing) and chemical (digestion) processes in order to break down food into its useful constituent parts (nutrients) and waste.

- **The endocrine system**, which produces and distributes hormones, the body's chemical communication system that governs the function of... well, pretty much everything.

- **The exocrine system**, which represents the parts of the body that are on the "outside", such as the skin, hair and nails, and includes the exocrine glands that are responsible for producing sweat.

- **The immune system**, which defends the body against foreign invaders, including those that can cause disease. It is also responsible for triggering and fighting allergic reactions, and includes many various and complex subsystems that exists within all parts of the body – including, for example, the skin and intestines.

- **The musculo-skeletal system**, which through the bones and muscles, provides the body with support and movement.

- **The nervous system**, which collects and processes information from our senses and brain, directing all other bodily processes and functions, including movement.

- **The renal system**, which filters the blood to produce waste products in the form of urine.

- **The reproductive system**, which works closely with the endocrine system in order to balance and produce the hormones that are essential to human reproduction.

- **The respiratory system**, which controls breathing and works closely with the cardiovascular system in the transport and transfer of oxygen throughout the body, and the removal of waste in the form of carbon dioxide.

- **The sensory system**, which works closely with the nervous system in order to pass sensory information to the brain.

All these systems require macro- and micronutrients in order to function optimally. Macronutrients are carbohydrates (which we need for energy), fats (which we need for hormone production and also for energy stores) and protein (which provides the building blocks of our cells), and micronutrients are all the vitamins, minerals, enzymes and so on that help to improve the health of the connective tissues in our body, cell structure, biochemical processes and myriad other functions that support the work of the main body systems. Oh, and not forgetting that we need water, too.

MACRO- AND MICRONUTRIENTS

Although nutrition itself is not the focus of this book, in order to understand why orthorexia – stripping certain nutrients from your diet – is unhealthy, it's important to have a basic understanding of what nutrients are and how they work on the body. This box summarises the macronutrients, while the main micronutrients are presented in the table overleaf. (There are many more; the table is just a snapshot.)

CARBOHYDRATE

The primary roles of carbohydrates in the diet include:

- Providing energy for physical activity
- Providing energy for the correct operation of organs
- Regulating blood-glucose levels for brain function
- Sparing the breakdown of protein for energy
- Preventing ketosis, which results from the breakdown of fats
- Providing good levels of fibre (in wholegrain foods) for a healthy gut

Good sources of carbohydrate include: whole grains, beans, pulses, potatoes, fruit, vegetables and dairy.

PROTEIN

Every cell in your body contains protein, so meeting your protein requirement is essential for your health. The primary roles of proteins in the diet include:

- Repairing and renewing body tissues and muscles
- Manufacturing hormones, including insulin

- Providing enzymes that bind to molecules to speed up chemical reactions within the body
- Supporting the immune system by helping the formation of antibodies to ward off invasion
- Providing energy when carbohydrate resources are low

Good sources of protein include: fish, poultry, eggs, meat, tofu, beans and pulses.

FATS

The primary roles of fats in the diet include:

- Providing an energy back-up system when carbohydrates are unavailable or depleted
- Supporting cell growth
- Protecting organs
- Providing the body with insulation
- Facilitating the absorption of fat-soluble vitamins (A, D, E, and K)
- Manufacturing some hormones

Good sources of essential fats include: olive and rapeseed oils, oily fish, avocados, seeds and nuts.

$\triangleright$

THE MAIN MICRONUTRIENTS

Mineral/ Vitamin	Used to support	Main dietary sources
Calcium	Bone health	Dairy, including milk, yogurt and cheese; soya milk and products; canned fish with bones
	Strong teeth	
	Muscle contraction	
	Cell signalling	
	Blood clotting	
	Nerve function	
Iron	Efficient transport of oxygen around the body	Red meat; eggs; plant foods such as green leafy vegetables, dried fruit, beans and pulses (Note that wholegrain cereals are not a key dietary source of fibre, unless you combine with vitamin C to improve absorption.)
Potassium	Nerve signalling	Bananas, citrus fruits, tomatoes; green leafy vegetables; beans and pulses
	Muscle function	
	Fluid balance	

▷

Mineral/ Vitamin	Used to support	Main dietary sources
Zinc	Immune health Healing wounds Cell repair	Meat; beans and pulses
Vitamin D	Immune health Mood Muscle recovery Bone health	Canned fish with bones; some fortified milks and margarines (Note that the body's primary source of vitamin D is sunlight.)
Vitamin C	Immune health Iron absorption Cell repair Healing wounds	Berry fruits, citrus fruits, tomatoes; potato skin
B-vitamins	Breakdown of energy from food Nervous system function Manufacturing red blood cells	Whole grains; green leafy vegetables; many fruits; eggs; meat and poultry

DIET: THE BOOK OF FOOD RULES

While orthorexia is a relatively newly identified eating disorder, diets and food trends have been around for years – it seems men and women have been looking at ways to perfect the body beautiful since time immemorial. However, there is definitely a shift in the way we think about what it means to have a healthy body and that's reflected in the trends we see in what constitutes healthy eating.

In the 1980s and 90s, when I was an impressionable teenager, it was all about being thin and getting that way by restricting calories. Diets such as the Rosemary Conley Hip & Thigh Diet, WeightWatchers and Slimming World (which all still exist today) focused on reducing daily calories, whether that was through restricting portion size or focusing on nutrient-rich but energy-stable (known as low-GI) foods. Even with these approaches, though, a dieter could still maintain a balanced nutritional intake of all food groups. In effect, as long as your energy intake was lower than your energy output, you would lose weight.

Today, happily we are more of the mindset that "thin" doesn't necessarily mean healthy or beautiful – this is a positive shift, and I welcome it (if you look at paintings of women over the course of history, you'll see that the fashion for what constitutes the body beautiful is cyclical – we just happen to be in a relatively good place in terms of body image and health right now). However, the knock-on effect in terms of diet trend isn't so positive. Today, the most popular diets are no longer to do with energy in and energy out, but the notion of nutritional purity. As we know, orthorexia is less about weight loss and more about "clean" eating – modern diet trends and orthorexia, then, go hand in hand.

So, if we aren't necessarily focusing on restricting calories, what are we doing? Modern diets and dietary fads tend to focus on removing individual ingredients or whole food groups because they are deemed to be harmful in some way. Detox, plant-based, sugar-free, gluten-free and low-carbohydrate/high-fat diets all provide "rules" that remove certain nutritional groups from the diet, often under the promise of some particular health benefit (and often that's not weight loss). And it's these rules that so appeal to anyone who is susceptible to orthorexia. To an orthorexic mind, following the rules to the letter (with a fundamental commitment equal to religious belief) represents positive behaviour, even when the effects are damaging.

There is one food rule, which occurs in diets by many different names, that seems to be most popular with those susceptible to orthorexia: eat fewer carbohydrates. Low-carbohydrate diets come in many different guises: a high-protein diet, such as the Dukan and Atkins diets, inevitably means restricting carbs; a high-fat diet (yes, high fat), such as the ketogenic diet, usually means low-carb; gluten-free and sugar-free diets – again, low-carb. Don't be fooled. These are the same wolf, he is just a master of disguise. When looking at the way in which an orthorexic is tempted into a diet regime or fad, it makes sense, then, to start with low-carb.

THE LOW-CARB DIET

Very low-carbohydrate diets, such as the ketogenic diet, permit only 50g of carbohydrate a day. To give you an idea of what that means in practice, one medium-sized baked potato with its skin contains approximately 50g of carbohydrate; a medium slice of wholemeal bread provides 15g. In effect, then, a person on such a restricted carbohydrate diet can eat only vegetables, cutting out all other carb sources – bread, pasta, rice, dairy and even fruit. Usually, the main source of nutrition then becomes fat, from foods such as cream, butter, coconut oil, nuts, avocados and higher-fat cuts of meat.

More moderate carb-restricted diets usually advocate around 150g of carbohydrate a day. This means that usually there is a significant reduction in the consumption of specific high-carb foods, such as bread, pasta and rice. Oats, sweet potato, quinoa and fruit are accepted in small quantities (perhaps at one to two meals a day); while refined and processed carbohydrates are a no-go at all. The remainder of the diet tends to be high in protein, and includes such foods as eggs, lean cuts of meat, and chicken and fish.

What's the promise?

Primarily, the promises of a low-carb diet are weight loss and blood-glucose management, particularly for those at risk of Type-II diabetes or heart disease, and those at risk of certain cancers.

Individuals who are susceptible to orthorexia, or who already have it, use the possibility of controlling potential long-term health problems, even when research links are tenuous, as a way of validating their obsessive carb restriction. Even those who have no underlying risk for disease or diabetes use the promise of reduced risk as the reason to control their diet.

On a slightly different note, many endurance athletes also favour low-carb as a way to eat. They hypothesize that removing carbohydrate from the diet forces the body to use fat for fuel, a limitless source of energy. As I've already covered, many individuals with orthorexia also have an unhealthy relationship with exercise. Training becomes an obsessive regime that exists even through pain or illness. Any possible suggestion that a change in diet could improve performance is another hook toward physical perfection and purity.

True or false gold?

The most compelling scientific evidence for following a very low-carbohydrate diet is that it can significantly improve the management of epilepsy. There is some emerging evidence that it can also help to improve blood-sugar stability and effectively maintain weight loss in those already diagnosed with Type-II diabetes. However, it is important to stress that there have been no longitudinal studies to confirm any of the ongoing benefits for very low-carb diets – in other words, while there may be positive effects in the short term, we don't yet know whether those effects are sustainable.

In a healthy diet, nutrition experts recommend that we eat a fist-sized portion of carbohydrate at every meal and that the carbohydrate should come from whole grains, beans, pulses, fruit, vegetables, milk and yogurts, rather than from processed and high-sugar sources, such as sweets, biscuits or white bread.

Interestingly, when it comes to weight loss, peer reviews suggest that there is no significant difference in weight loss over a period of two years between those who reduce their carb intake to less than 50g a day (very low) compared with those on a low-fat diet (low-fat diets tend to have normal or higher carbohydrate intakes). Looking at the body as a piece of biochemistry this makes sense – it's not the removal of a food group that results in weight loss, but the accompanying reduction in calories.

Compare two meals – one low in carbohydrate, one low in fat. Let's say your normal mid-week meal consists of steak, chips and peas. You decide to cut your carbs so you take out the chips, and perhaps even add a few extra peas to help fill you up. Even so, without a normal-sized portions of chips, your meal now has 250kcals fewer than it did when the chips were there.

Alternatively, you decide on a low-fat diet. So, instead of a mid-week portion of macaroni cheese, you have the equivalent bowl of pasta stirred through with a plain tomato and basil sauce – removing the high-fat cheese sauce and replacing it with a vegetable version will save you about 200kcals.

In this example, there is a slight net benefit of being on a low-carb diet, but remembering that we have to look at our nutrition over the course of weeks and months rather than days, overall weight loss is going to be roughly the same even when carbs are present and something else is missing.

As far as athletic performance goes, scientific studies presently conclude that a very low-carbohydrate diet does not improve performance, particularly when there is need for speed. The body uses carbohydrate as an immediate fuel source – so if your muscles need energy, carbohydrate is the best way to provide it. Converting fat to energy is a longer, inefficient process. For endurance athletes it is an important way to keep going, but for most of us thinking of fat as fuel is definitely false gold.

HIGH-FAT DIETS

There is much publicity about the weight-loss benefits of following a high-fat diet – and the food industry has jumped on the band wagon, providing many readily available high-fat options including coconut-based yogurts and other desserts. However, the type of fat you eat is key. A study in the *British Medical Journal* in 2016 concluded that when saturated fats (such as fats in butter, on meat, and in coconut oil) are replaced with polyunsaturated fats (such as the fats in avocado, olive and rapeseed oil, and nuts) and wholegrain carbohydrates or plant-based proteins, the risk of cardiovascular disease is significantly decreased. There is one exception, which is the saturated fat in dairy food. This seems to have no direct negative effect on cardiovascular health and may even have a protective factor. The point here is that eating high-fat options in general is not necessarily good for your health – understanding the nature of fats and the impact of different types of fat on the body is key.

In which case, unless you are very careful about the types of fat you eat, you don't fall into the trap of supermarket advertising, and you combine healthy fats with other nutrients to ensure you have a balanced diet, following a high-fat, low-carb diet in the long-term could have a detrimental effect on cardiovascular health, increasing your susceptibility to heart disease and heart attack.

Why is carbohydrate essential for health?

Carbohydrate is made up of sugars known as saccharides. These can be further subdivided as monosaccharides (made up of one carbohydrate molecule), disaccharides (two molecules), oligosaccharides (three to nine molecules) and polysaccharides (ten or more molecules).

Mono- and disaccharides are "simple" sugars, such as glucose (mono-), sucrose or cane sugar (di-). or lactose or milk sugar (di-). Oligosaccharides are fructo-oligosaccharides, such as the sugars in onions and artichokes, or galacto-oligosacchrides, such as in beans, peas, whole grains and cabbage. Polysaccharides occur in starch foods, including cereals, breads and pasta. Oligo- and polysaccharides are often referred to as complex carbohydrates.

So, how is this relevant to orthorexia? Well, the terminology "simple" and "complex" has led to a lot of misinformation. People often think that all simple carbohydrates are "bad". This is because they are assumed to release sugar quickly into the blood stream causing an instant rise in blood sugar, that leads to energy peaks and troughs and mood swings. Complex carbs on the other hand are all thought of as "good", because they are generically claimed to be slow-acting – they release sugar slowly into the blood stream, sustaining more stable blood-sugar levels. While type-casting carbohydrates in this way provides an easy classification system, it does little to represent the true nutritional quality of the different types in all their food forms – and that's dangerous for anyone susceptible to an eating disorder.

First, not all simple carbohydrates are created equal. The fruit sugar fructose, for example, is found in fruit and is actually slow to release sugar into the blood, as well as being found in foods that are nutrient-dense (in other words, fruit contains simple carbs and is good for you!) On the other hand, refined complex carbohydrates, such as those found in white bread and pasta, raise blood sugar rapidly and are nutritionally quite poor.

How quickly we digest a food and assimilate its nutrients into our body is determined by a variety of factors, including the combination of nutrients in the food. When you consume carbohydrate, whether you have protein with it (a white-bread tuna sandwich, say) and whether you eat the whole fruit or just the juice (a whole apple, or a glass of apple juice) will have an impact on the way the sugars act on your body. Protein and fibre slow down the release of sugar. Indeed, preparation comes into it, too: juicing fruit – which removes the skin and begins the process of breaking down the cell walls in the fruit – creates a drink that causes a sharp rise in blood glucose.

Beans, pulses and vegetables are also high in fibre, making them hard for the body to digest quickly. They don't then contribute to the body's energy store and they raise blood sugar only slowly. There's no need to avoid carbohydrate in these foods, because they are filling (so you don't feel hungry again too quickly, reducing your likelihood of snacking) and nutritionally dense.

We've just blasted a popular myth favoured by so many pseudo-nutritionists and celebrity dieters: that carbohydrates cause weight gain so they are bad for us. No, they aren't. The right carbohydrates, eaten in the right way at the right time in healthy amounts, are an essential component of a healthy diet and a healthy body.

What is the right amount?

Reference intake guidelines in the UK recommend 300g carbohydrate a day for an average-weight adult man and 260g for an average-weight adult woman, if he or she is doing a moderate amount of exercise (say 60 minutes three or four times a week) and wanting to maintain weight within a healthy range for his or her height. These values are generally lower in the USA, and will vary from country to country, so it's worth checking with your medical practitioner what's recommended where you live – culture, climate and lifestyle all affect our eating patterns as individual populations.

If your body has enough carbohydrate to meet its immediate energy requirements, and the body's glycogen stores are full, any extra carbohydrate is stored as fat. However, let's not give carbohydrate all the bad press: the body turns any additional energy coming from the diet – whether that's from carbohydrate, protein or fat – into glucose and then stores it as fat. This process is not specific to carbs.

CARBS AND YOUR BODY

The primary role of carbohydrate is to provide your body with energy. Your body prefers glucose as its energy source above all other, so when you eat carbs that's the first thing your body makes from it. You might think in that case, given that you aren't an athlete or exercise only moderately, that makes glucose a non-essential nutrient for your particular lifestyle. Think again.

Unless you are undergoing a period of prolonged starvation, glucose is virtually the only fuel your body uses to feed your brain. The brain lacks fuel stores of its own. As a result every day it consumes about 120g of glucose – the equivalent of an energy input of about 420kcals. Put another way, when your body is at rest, your brain is using about 60 per cent of your average daily glucose intake.

WHY DOES THE BODY NEED CARBS?

The brain is an exceptionally concentrated area of nerve cells. Known as neurons, these brain cells use glucose from your diet to fuel their cellular activities. If glucose levels are low within the brain, it can't produce neurotransmitters (the brain's

▷

chemical messengers). This results in a breakdown of communication between neurons, meaning in turn that the messages that tell our body or mind what to do or how to focus don't get through – it's as if they fall down the gap in a broken bridge. Most of us have experienced what this feels like at some time or another – think about how you lose concentration or find it hard to make decisions when your sugar-levels are low. For someone with orthorexia who has removed the brain's source of fuel from their diet, brain function quickly feels impaired.

In desperation, your body looks for back-up. If you starve your brain of glucose it signals to the liver to help out. First, the liver releases stored glycogen (converted excess glucose), but those stores aren't limitless: if you aren't eating carbohydrate, they will eventually run out, too. Dutifully, the hormone glucogen steps in to help the liver work out what's going on and how to respond. Glucogen sends a signal to your liver that circulating glucose/glycogen levels are too low and it needs to send up some emergency fuel supplies. In response, the liver converts stored fat into ketones – these provide the emergency brain

▷

fuel. If you rely on ketones for too long, though, you are likely to experience dizziness, headaches and lack of concentration. We need more research to determine the long-term negative effects of ketone use, but circumstantial evidence in cases of anorexia tells us that brain function suffers when the brain has only ketones for food.

BUT WHAT ABOUT THE REST OF YOUR BODY?

Insufficient carbohydrate stores (either because you aren't eating enough of them in the first place, or because you are eating recommended amounts, but then exercising a lot and not replenishing the stores) leads your body to look for alternative sources for energy. Usually those sources are protein and body (muscle) tissue. However, proteins are needed for essential other work in the body: building cells (including muscle cells), maintaining and repairing muscle, and looking after other body tissue, including skin, hair and nails. Once protein stores run out, the body breaks down its own tissue as fuel – that's when you get into the realms of muscle wastage. Starving your body of carbohydrate, therefore, has a detrimental effect not just on your brain, but on all your body tissues.

▷

Finally, research on athletes who restrict their carbohydrate intake is showing links between very low carbohydrate intake and immune suppression. Many athletes who don't have sufficient immediate energy supply suffer from recurring infections, particularly after a high-intensity training block. In more severe cases, carb restriction affects athletes at a biochemical level, resulting in over-training syndrome, from which it can take years to recover and may even end a sporting career.

Micronutrients and carbs

We've already established that carbohydrate is a macronutrient – along with fat and protein, it is one of the "big three" essential nutrients for the body. However, carb foods also contain myriad micronutrients – vitamins and minerals that are also essential to health (see table, pages 55–6).

For example, many wholegrain and complex carbohydrates are high in B-vitamins, which your body needs to release energy from its food, as well as for blood, brain and nerve health. Dried fruit, beans and pulses provide iron, an essential mineral involved in the uptake and transport of oxygen around the body. Milk and yogurt are not only good sources of carbohydrate, they are also high in calcium, which is essential for good muscle contraction, nerve signalling and bone health.

DAIRY-FREE DIETS AND BONE HEALTH

It's not unusual for those suffering from orthorexia to add one dietary restriction to another in a cumulative effect. The result is to increasingly limit permitted foods in the pursuit of a purity that never comes. One combination I often see in my clinic is adding dairy-free to low-carb – this proves a dangerous combo for bone health and illustrates how all nutrients work together for optimum health.

Many low-carb diets are naturally high in animal protein, as this provides the body with an alternative, filling source of energy. However, high-protein diets lower the pH (the relative levels of acid and alkaline) of the body to slightly acidic. In itself, this isn't too much of a problem – your clever body releases calcium ions from your bone to neutralize the acid, restoring acid–alkaline balance. However, if you are on a dairy-free diet, your body is probably not meeting its daily calcium requirements, which means

$\triangleright$

that your bone cannot replace what it has lost. Over time, your bones become weaker, increasing your risk of stress fractures and even osteoporosis (a bone-wasting disease).

How far is too far?

I like – and welcome – the idea that we educate ourselves about the good and bad of everything we eat. For most of us, we hear where the dangers lie, we log them, and perhaps we become more mindful – making minor, positive adjustments to our diet for our overall health and well-being, but we don't become a slave to them.

For someone suffering from orthorexia, however, the negative messages are all-consuming. Carbohydrates are bad for us, and low-carb represents clean-eating (improved health and well-being), so we must stick to the dietary rules at all times and at all costs.

Here are some of the early warning signs that reducing carbs has gone too far:

- **Lethargy and fatigue** – the body may feel like you are wading through treacle.

- **Pear-drop aroma on the breath**, which can quickly turn into halitosis. These changes occur as a side-effect of ketone production.

- **Constipation** – insufficient carbohydrate foods in the diet usually means reduced dietary fibre, too (whole grains, cereals, beans and pulses are all important sources of fibre in the diet). Constipation is itself a sign that your digestive tract is in trouble and recent studies have indicated that high-fibre carbohydrates have an important role to play in optimizing the gut microbiome, which itself is an essential part of the immune system and helps prevent obesity.

- **Recurrent dizziness, headaches and lack of concentration** – low blood-glucose levels over time affect the functioning of the nervous system.

- **Lowered libido, bone weakness and absence of menstruation** – prolonged carb restriction can interfere with the body's ability to produce sex hormones in both men and women. Not only does this affect libido, but also impairs bone density. In women, the affect on the sex hormones can cause intermittent periods, or result in no periods at all (amenorrhoea).

- **Low mood** – there are numerous studies that have linked very low carbohydrate intakes with low mood and depression. The exact mechanism for this is unclear, but it is thought that lowered carbohydrate intake impairs the production of serotonin, our natural anti-depressant.

- **Poor sleep patterns** – the body needs carbohydrate to manufacture the "sleep hormone" tryptophan, so some low-carb dieters complain of poor sleep. There is a knock-on effect of this, too, because when we don't sleep properly we have reduced energy levels and are more susceptible to low mood.

THE TRUTH ABOUT HIGH-PROTEIN DIETS

As we've already established, high-protein diets are just low-carb by a different name (pasta and potatoes make way for fish, lean meat, eggs and other high-protein foods as a means to fill us up), so they carry with them all the pitfalls of any other low-carb diet. Nonetheless, sold as high-protein they also come with their own particular apparent benefits. The greatest of these are weight loss and increased muscle mass – body-builders and weight-trainers are the biggest champions and, in the next chapter, I'll talk about how this particular demographic has influenced orthorexia.

The theory goes that protein provides the building blocks of the body's muscle (and other tissue). Therefore, if the body has more protein, it has more blocks with which to build a bigger physical structure. The more lean muscle mass we have, the less body fat. This, in turn, increases our metabolic rate, because muscle speeds up metabolism, burning calories even during rest. By comparison, on traditional calorie-counting weight-loss strategies, you lose both fat and muscle, which means that at some point your metabolism will slow down and plateau, making further weight loss more difficult to achieve. Alongside this, high-protein foods have a high satiety, helping you to feel fuller for longer. If you feel full up, you're less likely to snack, which means you're overall more likely to consume fewer calories.

▷

DO THEY WORK?

As always, it's not that simple. At first, a high-protein diet combined with anabolic exercise such as weight-training will build muscle mass. But studies show that, over time, even though a seasoned body-builder might need a bit more protein than you or me, he or she certainly doesn't need anything like the amounts at the start of the process. In fact, once the body has reached a new state of homeostasis (balance), it's more likely that excess protein will be being stored as fat than as muscle. Basically, the body adapts to the demands of training.

It's also worth stating that eating protein alone does not in itself magically build muscle. In fact, you'd need to lift weights three to five times a week for at least 12 weeks to have any discernible change in your body composition. Plus, restricting carbs at the expense of protein in fact results in reduced muscle mass. Without carbs the body's ability to produce the hormone insulin is reduced, and without insulin the body can't build muscle. It seems, then, that on balance a high-protein diet combined with low carbs with the aim of becoming leaner and stronger is something of a myth.

HOW MUCH PROTEIN DO WE REALLY NEED?

A balanced diet, with a little of everything, will usually provide just the right amount of protein for good health. Guidelines suggest that the average (70kg) man needs about 55–70g protein a day; while the average (60kg) woman about 48–60g (the formula is 0.8–1g protein for every 1kg bodyweight). And, the body uses that protein best when it's served alongside some carbohydrate. So, think:

- a jacket potato with tuna (half a can of tuna provides about 10g protein)
- a card-pack-sized portion of chicken with a fistful of rice (about 20g protein)
- two eggs on toast (about 12g of protein)

You get the picture.

GOING GLUTEN-FREE

We've already established that a gluten-free diet is a low-carb diet by another name. However, it needs special mention, because of course there are circumstances when following a gluten-free diet is essential to health. In the orthorexic mind, this genuine health reason becomes the perfect excuse to follow food rules to the point of obsession.

Gluten is the protein found within wheat and related grains, including barley and rye. Therefore, it's a constituent of foods such as bread, pasta and cereals, of many pre-packed foods such as burgers and sausages (because they often contain breadcrumbs), and of drinks such as beer and whisky.

The gluten-free epidemic

In recent years there has been a lot written about the effects of gluten on the body – with many people blaming it for symptoms such as bloating, fatigue and joint pain – leading to a significant trend toward "going gluten-free". Retailers and manufacturers have picked up on this: even foods, such as rice, yogurts, dried fruits, that are naturally gluten-free now appear in packaging shouting as much; I've even seen body lotion labelled "gluten-free". Many high-profile individuals, including athletes, celebrities and food bloggers, have reported health and performance benefits since removing gluten from their diets; some have even gone as far as to say that it has cured illness, particularly auto-immune conditions, such as rheumatoid arthritis, sarcoidosis, thyroid disease and so on. The hypothesis goes that gluten causes inflammation in the body, and that this inflammation in turn leads to the immune system attacking the cells in its own body.

Finally, many claim that because the digestive system finds it hard to break down gluten in food, gluten in the diet makes it hard to lose weight. In which case, the theory is that removing gluten leads to weight loss.

True or false gold?

Although it is true that the body finds it harder to break down gluten than it does other forms of protein, healthy bodies are perfectly able to do so with the body absorbing and utilizing the gluten as necessary. There is no scientific evidence to suggest that there are necessarily any benefits to following a gluten-free diet unless you have a medical reason (see box, pages 82–3) to do so. Claims that those following a gluten-free diet feel less bloated and healthier *are* probably true – but it's not necessarily the gluten that's been the problem. If you cut down on refined and processed carbohydrates to within guideline levels (remembering that most of us eat far too much white bread and pasta anyway), you will feel "lighter".

We all have the tendency to be easily led – but the orthorexic mind is especially suggestible when it comes to any dietary approach for which there are claims of purifying the body. Gluten-free, with all the hype and advertising, immediately appeals: "If it's in the news, if so-and-so is doing it, if it's highlighted on packaging, it must be good for me." However, don't be fooled into thinking that a gluten-free diet is necessarily healthier than a diet that allows gluten. Gluten-free products tend to be lacking in whole grains, which (for example) provide B-vitamins and fibre (it's possible to have wholegrain gluten-free), and also to be higher in fat and sugar, in order to make them more palatable.

COELIAC DISEASE

The only auto-immune condition that truly requires a gluten-free diet is coeliac disease. This disease occurs when eating gluten triggers the immune system to attack the lining of the small intestine, damaging it to the extent that it becomes unable to absorb vital nutrients such as calcium, iron and carbohydrate from food. The symptoms of coeliac disease are usually weight loss, extreme fatigue (as a result of iron deficiency), bloating, and very frequent bowel movements. Poor calcium levels

▷

mean that those who have coeliac disease may be at an increased risk of osteoporosis. The only treatment for the disease that we know of is to avoid gluten altogether. As soon as a person has been given a medical diagnosis, he or she will immediately be advised to adopt a gluten-free diet, which they will have to follow for life. In this case, going gluten-free is genuinely essential for good health.

Gluten-free and weight loss

We know that orthorexia primarily focuses on perfect health rather than weight loss. Nonetheless, claims for weight loss abound when it comes to advocating gluten-free diets, so it it's worth just looking at where these claims come from and why – and whether or not they are well founded.

Advocates of gluten-free diets argue that gluten upsets the gut microbiome – the delicate balance of gut flora that form an essential part of our gut health and immune system. There is emerging, tentative evidence that an unhealthy microbiome leads to weight gain. However, keeping the microbiome optimal is not all down to whether or not we eat gluten – there are many nutritional factors at play, including the inclusion of whole grains, many of which contain gluten, which are an important source of prebiotics. The body uses prebiotics to feed probiotics – another name for gut flora – so that they can colonize our guts and create an optimal environment for health.

However, gluten-free diets do tend to result in weight loss – so, why? The answer is simple – for all the reasons that any low-carb diet will result in weight loss: it's the removal of calories, rather than the removal of gluten that's working.

Gluten-free and the dangers for health

It's worth remembering that in the orthorexic mind becoming gluten-free is one way to achieve a state of physiological purity. A gluten-free diet presents a perfect opportunity for rule-setting; for exercising the need for control. However, while the body doesn't need gluten itself for good health, there are lots of other nutrients in foods that contain gluten that the body does need.

Let's take an example. Many champions of the gluten-free diet encourage the use of spiralized vegetables in place of spaghetti – even in place of gluten-free spaghetti. While I am a great fan of vegetables, they don't provide everything we need for health. Let's compare:

- One 140g cooked serving of wholewheat gluten-free spaghetti provides 38g of carbohydrate, 7.5g protein, 0.8g fat and 6.3g fibre. It also provides 8 per cent of our daily iron and is a great source of all the B-vitamins except B12 (which is found only in animal products).

- In comparison, a similar-sized portion of spiralized vegetables provides 10g carbohydrate, no protein, no fat and 2g fibre. It provides no iron at all and a very small percentage of vitamin B6 (and none of the other B-vitamins).

While someone suffering from orthorexia might feel virtuous because he or she has removed the gluten, and therefore the carbohydrate, in fact the net result is to have starved the body of significant amounts of other nutrients that are essential for good health. A spiralized meal might mean we feel full on the veg for a short time, but the body will soon catch up. Messages will go to the brain that it needs more food – and then one of two things is likely to happen:

- We might ignore the signals, but berate ourselves for feeling hungry and feel that somehow we have "failed" in the quest to follow the rules properly, perpetuating the cycle of negative self-image.

- Or, we might give in to the hunger, have a snack and then – again – berate ourselves that we have failed in the quest to follow the rules.

Both outcomes set up a cycle of negative emotion, which can only, in turn, exacerbate orthorexia altogether.

REALITY CHECK: BLOATING AND GLUTEN

It's very easy to lay the blame for bloating at the door of gluten. I have seen so many individuals in my clinic who have self-diagnosed gluten (or eating foods such as pasta) for being the reason they feel bloated and uncomfortable. My instinct in these cases is to press for more information, which often reveals that it's portion size that's the problem – not what's in the meal itself. For every 1g of pasta you eat, your body holds up to 4g of fluid – the maths is really simple. The solution is simple, too: reduce

▷

portion size and if you want to feel you're eating a bit more, top up with spiralized vegetables – that way you get balanced benefit from the carbohydrate food, and a few different vitamins (such as vitamin C) from the veg.

How far is too far?

As I've said, in moderation reducing carb intake is not necessarily detrimental to good health. So, how do we know when things have gone too far? When spaghetti always becomes spiralized vegetables and lettuce leaves always replace bread wraps or sandwiches, I think it's time to take stock and consider what's driving the changes on your plate (assuming, that is, that there is no medical reason to remove gluten from the diet).

If we take a step back in the chronology, it's also worth looking out for a slide into this: what might have started as a more balanced carb-checked diet (eating more wholegrain carbohydrate, say, rather than refined carbs), then becomes low-carb, which then becomes gluten-free. Once this slide into nutritional restriction is out of control and begins to interfere with day-to-day living and decision-making, it is no longer the sufferer who is controlling their diet, but the diet that is controlling the sufferer. The irony is that the need to achieve purity through strict dietary control has in fact had the opposite effect. The results can be significant nutritional deficiency and physical illness associated with all disordered eating. (Please bear in mind if you know someone on a gluten-free diet in this stage of illness, needing to be gluten-free becomes a self-fulfilling prophecy – without having digested gluten for a long time, the body "forgets" how to do it. Any reintroduction into the diet needs to be slow and measured to give the body time to readapt.)

SUGAR-FREE DIET

If I could pick one food ingredient about which there is most confusion and misinformation, it would be sugar. In recent years, sugar has become the new scapegoat for poor health, being blamed for the rise in obesity and Type-II diabetes. I've always been a little sceptical about demonizing just one food ingredient for a whole population epidemic. Studies show that, in fact, obesity is a multi-factorial disease and being overweight or obese can increase your risk of developing Type-II diabetes, but it is not an inevitability.

Sugar-free diets, themselves a version of a low-carb diet, come in several shapes and sizes. Some diets recommend removing added sugar (so, cutting out foods that do not naturally contain sugar but have it added); while others are more extreme and advocate removing all refined sugar. This basically means removing any white (processed) carbohydrate, including table sugar, and products or meals made using white pasta, rice, bread and flour. The diet replaces refined sugar with natural sugars, such as maple syrup, honey, molasses, and coconut sugar. Processed white carbohydrates are replaced with products made using spelt or wholegrain flours – we see them in the shops as wholegrain bread and pasta, for example.

The promises of a sugar-free diet

Sugar-free diets promise purity of health that shows in clear skin, bright eyes and luscious locks. Furthermore, advocates claim that reducing sugar will optimize weight and energy levels, and slow down the effects of ageing.

So, where do these claims come from? Eating refined sugar does cause your blood-sugar levels to spike and dip, putting pressure on your body's manufacture of insulin, the hormone that balances blood-sugar levels in the body. Remember that when the body releases insulin, it uses excess glucose as its immediate fuel store, then squirrels away any leftover glucose as fat. For this reason, sugar in the diet is held responsible for weight gain.

Furthermore, sugar-free advocates claim that refined sugar is almost addictive – some have suggested that eating sugar leads to cravings for more sugar. The more you eat, the more you crave, leading to excess. The natural alternatives to white sugar are thought to have a slower release of glucose into the body, and in addition provide the body with additional minerals and vitamins.

Finally, advocates claim that excess glucose in the system binds to the "youth" proteins in the skin, turning them brittle and therefore contributing to the signs of ageing.

True or false gold?

A 2015 report by the UK's Scientific and Advisory Committee on Nutrition (SACN) determined that "added" or "free" sugar should make up no more than 5 per cent of an average adult's total energy intake, to a maximum of 30g a day.

This recommendation is based on SACN's assessment of the ways in which free sugars demonstrably and measurably increase the risk of dental caries and their effects on total energy intake. In general, a higher intake of free sugar increases the risk of an overall higher intake of energy, in turn increasing the likelihood that we will end up eating more calories than guidelines recommend. That, in turn again, leads to increased likelihood of obesity. Reduce sugar intake, on the other hand, and the problem starts to fade away.

It's important to make clear that the findings were looking at consumption of refined sugar, not sugar that is naturally found in fruit (known as fructose) or milk (lactose). These are "intrinsic" sugars and are actually the only "natural" forms of sugar.

"Free" sugars include:

- white table sugar
- brown sugar
- honey
- maple syrup
- agave syrup
- coconut sugar
- molasses

- date syrup
- high fructose corn syrup

What is interesting is that those who endorse a refined-sugar-free lifestyle for health benefits often promote the use of maple syrup, honey, date syrup, and coconut sugar as acceptable alternatives. They claim that these plant sugars are better for us, because they not only contain additional minerals, they also release energy at a slower rate than table sugar, thereby stabilizing blood-sugar levels and helping us to feel more satisfied for longer. And here we have yet more false gold.

Let's first look at the labels "refined" and "unrefined". The term refined is defined as the removal of unwanted elements or impurities by processing. In the context of food, this doesn't automatically make the resulting foodstuff unhealthy. Think of this in straightforward terms: if you were to eat an apple without its skin, although the apple wouldn't have all the nutrients it could provide because the skin has been removed, it's not *unhealthy* – there's still plenty of worthwhile nourishment in the flesh and core.

Furthermore, it's a red herring to think that refined white sugar is really any different to maple syrup that comes in a bottle. White sugar is extracted from the sugarcane plant; maple syrup is extracted from the sap of the maple tree. When we consume them, the body treats both types of processed sugar in exactly the same way. And, in a final irony, the main component of maple syrup is actually sucrose – white sugar. While I do think the body is an absolutely amazing machine, it doesn't have the ability to identify the original source of the sugar in its system – sugar is sugar. If you over-consume maple syrup it is no better for you than if you over-consume white sugar from sugarcane.

But, what about the claims for additional minerals and glowing skin? It's true that maple syrup has a slightly higher composition of magnesium, but this is significant for your body only if you are intending to eat 100g of maple syrup rather than 100g of white sugar – neither of which I advise you to do.

Finally, there is little evidence to suggest that one particular food, whether that's sugar or green beans, can have a drastically positive or negative effect on appearance. Your overall nutritional intake, as well as your exposure to the sun, and your levels of hydration, physical activity and stress, and very importantly your genetic make-up, all contribute to the appearance of your skin.

Sugar-free diets are misleading in so many ways. They give a false impression of what sugar is and the relative healthiness of one type of sugar over another. For orthorexics who remove sugar from their diet with an obsessive degree of rule-following, all the perils of a low-carb diet (remembering that sugar-free is low-carb by a different name) ensue: extreme fatigue, poor concentration and sleep, and hormonal and bone health disturbances, among others. Psychologically, what starts out as cutting down on fizzy drinks and sweets (and I agree that we could all do with cutting down on these) becomes panic about the amount of fruit sugar in a processed fruit yogurt (the benefits of protein and calcium far outweigh any potential spike in blood sugar from refined sugar in the yogurt). When you start looking for sugar, you see that it's everywhere. To aim to eradicate it is to drive an obsessive–compulsive conviction that results in overall nutritional deficit, not physiological purity.

REFINED CARBOHYDRATE: FACT AND FICTION

In a sugar-free diet, the rules remove refined carbohydrates and one question clients frequently ask me is, are refined carbohydrates really that bad

▷

for us? The simple answer is no; eaten in moderation they are not bad for us – it's the amount of them that we eat that can become a problem.

Pasta made from white flour from durum wheat is not highly processed, so while it is refined (because the flour is white), it is still relatively nutritious. Similarly white rice has had its husk, bran and germ removed which changes the flavour and reduces dietary fibre, but the rice still provides the body with carbohydrate, protein, minerals and vitamins.

The only exception to this rule is white bread, but I'm not talking about a freshly made loaf of white bread; I'm talking more about the sliced white you can buy in supermarkets. This is a product that has been very highly processed and provides very little nutritional value.

As a dietitian, I wholeheartedly encourage individuals to eat more wholegrain versions of foods in order to meet their fibre requirements for the day, but I also don't demonize white versions. Remember that how you cook a carbohydrate, or what you serve it with, also influences the body's

▷

ability to absorb and use it. While the sugars in white rice may be absorbed slightly more quickly than those in wholegrain, if I eat white rice with my favourite Thai red vegetable curry, the higher fat content of the curry slows down the glucose absorption anyway.

Sugar-free diet and the orthorexic mindset

As we have seen, the body needs a relatively regular supply of carbohydrate to work efficiently, and the need is especially relevant to the proper functioning of your brain (see pages 69–71).

However, popular culture, which demonizes sugar so readily, is far more in keeping with the orthorexic mindset. While there is no physiological need for free sugar in the diet, it is important to stress that even the SACN guidelines suggest that it can make up 5 per cent of total daily energy intake. If we are talking about rules, then there is no scientific rule that states there is no place for refined sugar in the diet. Nor is the "5 per cent" value a strict limit – it is a guideline on daily intake, but a little bit more on one day won't be the end of the world. The guidelines are there just to give us a sense of what falls within healthy parameters so that we don't consistently over-consume. Occasional indulgence is fine.

PLANT-BASED DIETS

So far we've looked at all the various guises for a low-carbohydrate diet – which, in whatever form it comes, is the number-one "rule" among orthorexics. But, if low-carb is the first rule, then eating only plant foods is the close second.

So much media hype tells us that we eat too much meat, too much dairy, and too few vegetables. The net result is that many people have come to associate a higher intake of fruit and vegetables with a healthier, purer body. Some studies tell us that increasing our intake of fruit and vegetables will help to protect us from certain diseases. All this is true, but – as always – it's not quite as black and white as the hype makes out.

What is a plant-based diet?

A plant-based diet is any diet that follows the rules of vegetarian or vegan ways of eating. For example, a plant-based diet could be:

- **Vegan** – excludes all animal products, which means meat, seafood, poultry, eggs and dairy.

- **Raw food vegan** – as vegan, but also excluding all foods cooked at temperatures greater than 48°C/118°F.

- **Lacto-vegetarian** – excludes eggs, meat, seafood and poultry, but includes milk products.

- **Ovo-vegetarian** – excludes meat, seafood, poultry and dairy products, but includes eggs.

- **Lacto-ovo vegetarian** – excludes meat, seafood and poultry, but includes eggs and dairy products.

In recent years some food and health bloggers have further tightened the rules of plant-based eating, advocating that a plant-based diet should comprise only "whole" plant foods, that is those free from artificial preservatives, colours, flavours, sweeteners and hydrogenated fats, and should be free from refined sugar.

Why do the rules appeal?

Remember that the orthorexic mind is looking for body purity. The rules of plant-based diets are hugely appealing on that front not only because a diet high in plant foods is claimed to be better for health (in particular in the prevention of cardiovascular disease and in lowering the risk of Type-II diabetes and obesity), but also because avoiding animal meat and products is perceived as ethically pure. Furthermore, harvesting vegetables is cheaper and more environmentally friendly, on balance, than producing meat. Nonetheless, ethical values are no excuse for eating unhealthily – it's perfectly possible to be healthy and to eat sustainably and with respect for animal welfare.

True or false gold?

There is a lot of evidence to suggest that a diet rich in fruit and vegetables and other plant foods (such as beans and pulses) can be beneficial to health, which is why government recommendations in developed countries are encouraging us to move from five- to eight-a-day, and in general to increase our intake of fruit, veg, beans, pulses, grains, nuts and seeds. However, this does not necessarily mean following a diet that is exclusively plant-based.

In the USA, researchers are trialling the notion of following a predominantly plant-based diet as a low-cost, low-risk exercise in managing chronic illness. They are hoping that it will reduce the amount of medication doctors have to prescribe to individuals who suffer with Type-II diabetes, cardiovascular disease, high blood pressure, and obesity.

My own research tells me that there are many medical references that associate vegetarianism and veganism with lower BMI (body mass index) and fewer incidents of the health problems associated with being overweight. However, what I see in my clinic tells me a slightly different story. In my practice, I come across individuals who have switched to vegetarianism or veganism in the name of improving their health and fitness, but for whom that has led to poor nutritional choices. For example, rather than eating meat or fish for protein, they might substitute high-fat, high-salt cheese. A vegan might substitute butter with nut oils and nut butters, which are very high in fat and calories. The result of these poor substitutions can lead to weight gain. Again, it's simple energy in and energy out.

EATING LA DOLCE VITA

As an interesting aside, the healthiest athletes I tend to see are usually those eating according to Mediterranean principles, which naturally includes

▷

a high percentage of plant-based foods in the form of vegetables and fruits, as well as fish rather than meat, and rapeseed and olive oil rather than butter. Incidentally, a Mediterranean diet also tends to include carbohydrate.

Undertaking a truly healthy plant-based diet is not just about cutting out all animal products. It requires education and then careful planning (weekly meal plans and shopping lists are a must, at least at the start) to ensure that the body gains the right amounts of protein, iron, calcium and B12 to meet its needs. All these nutrients are hard to find in a purely plant-based diet – you have to seek them out (see box, pages 103–4).

Trends for orthorexia

I would love to be able to write that recent fashion for plant-based diets is because we have become more aware of animal welfare and are making the choice to switch from eating meat for ethical reasons. However, I use the word "fashion" quite deliberately. Vegetarianism and veganism are popular because we have had a recent surge of media bloggers and even celebrities who have claimed it as a cure-all for human illness.

I want to be very clear that I am not anti-vegetarian nor anti-vegan: in fact, I have been vegetarian since I was 13 years old. Partly this is a result of my upbringing – my parents are of Indian heritage and they brought me up with a predominantly plant-based diet. A staple evening meal was dahl and rice, or chapati and chickpea and vegetable curry. My parents did not insist that I followed a strict vegetarian diet, but my mum never cooked meat, fish or poultry. She did serve up eggs, yogurt, milk and cheese for variety. While I was offered meat and fish at school and at friends' houses, I never particularly liked the taste or texture of them. By the time I was 13, I felt very uncomfortable about the slaughter of animals as a food source and so decided to become fully, consciously vegetarian. I guess because of my upbringing, I have always naturally understood how to make vegetarianism a balanced way to eat and I have never suffered with the nutritional deficiencies, such as low levels of iron, B12 and calcium, that are often associated with a vegetarian diet. Every now and again I do toy with the idea of becoming vegan, but I love cheese, yogurt and butter too much.

For me, plant-based eating is not a way to restrict or control my diet in the name of purity or optimal health. I take care to ensure that I meet my nutritional requirements and, while I naturally avoid meat, fish and poultry, that is where the restrictions stop. I prefer to make most of my meals from scratch if possible, but if on the odd occasion I have to use a readymade pasta sauce or shop-bought pizza, then I will. I may add extra vegetables and pulses to the meal to improve the nutritional quality. This is the difference between someone who has a healthy approach to plant-based eating and someone who uses the food rules as a method of control and restriction.

NUTRIENT GAPS IN A PLANT-BASED DIET

There are some key nutrients that both vegetarians and vegans need to take special care to seek out. With the exception of tofu, plant-based proteins are not "complete" – that is, they don't contain all the eight amino acids that the body needs for repair and regeneration. This means that, first and foremost, plant-based eaters need to make sure they consume a variety of vegetables and pulses, in combination, to get all the amino acids they need. Beans on toast or rice and lentils or quinoa and chickpeas are all good combos.

Plant-based diets are also low in iron, but the problem is exacerbated by the fact that they are also relatively high in phytates, antioxidant compounds

▷

that block the body's ability to absorb iron. One way to improve iron absorption from the foods that are available is to eat them with a source of vitamin C (so follow up a meal immediately with a glass of freshly pressed orange juice, for example).

One nutrient that is completely deficient in vegan diets is vitamin B12, which is found only in foods of animal origin and without which a person will start to experience symptoms such as pins and needles and specific forms of anaemia. Vegetarians can get B12 from eggs, milk and cheese, albeit in small quantities; vegans need to supplement.

Finally, calcium is hard to come by in a vegan diet (vegetarians who consume sufficient dairy should be fine). I recommend supplementation, because even foods that carry the name milk, cream or yogurt but are made using, say, coconut milk, are not rich sources of calcium, which is essential for bone health.

The slide into orthorexia

In the orthorexic mind what might start out as a claim for healthy eating slides into increasingly restrictive dietary rules. When it comes to plant-based diets, this slide is easy to map if you're looking out for it.

- First, the dieter removes red meat.

- Next, goes poultry and fish.

- Then, eggs and dairy disappear.

- Then, plant foods need to become "whole foods" and anything shop-bought or readymade disappears.

- Finally, everything has to be unrefined, or sugar free.

When people come to see me in the clinic and tell me they are vegan, I ask lots of questions – when I hear that soya milk has been replaced with almond milk (remember: expensive water) and that desserts aren't allowed because of the sugar in them, I have to ask myself whether I'm talking to someone with serious, ethical reasons for being so strictly vegan and a lot of naivety about nutrition; or someone who has tipped over, whose obsession with what goes into his or her body constitutes an eating disorder.

Veganism, in particular, has become a guise for disordered eating, including for orthorexia. Of course, I am definitely not saying that every single vegan has an eating disorder; just that veganism provides the perfect excuse for following food rules that result in the removal of whole food groups. There is much evidence to suggest that many individuals with an eating disorder become vegetarian or vegan during the early stages of their decline into the illness.

THE CASE OF JORDAN YOUNGER

One fairly high-profile example of how plant-based eating can actually become harmful is the case of Jordan Younger. In 2013, Jordan started The Blonde Vegan blog, sharing her healthy vegan recipes and photos. The blog became very popular very quickly, but just a year after she had started writing it, she made a confession: her restrictive diet was actually proving detrimental to her health and that was the complete opposite of the image she had wanted to portray. What had started out as a plant-based diet had soon spiralled into juice cleanses, and the removal of all processed or "refined" foods, including sugar, and white pasta and bread. She admitted that although she had been posting pictures of her "delicious and wholesome juices", the reality was they were making her sick. She was selling a lifestyle but actually not "feeling" it herself. She confessed to having orthorexia. While she was praised by many for bringing attention to this topic, she also instantly lost 1,000 of her followers for betraying her vegan lifestyle and roots. She has written about her experiences on her blog and in her book, *Breaking Vegan*.

THE DETOX DIET

Finally, this chapter wouldn't be complete unless we look at the role of detox diets in the orthorexic psyche. Although detox diets don't tend to remove single food groups, they do restrict overall calorie intake – and they come with a set of rules in the name of body purity (detox = detoxification; removing toxins) that can be deeply appealing to someone who is susceptible to eating disorders, including and especially orthorexia.

A detox diet aims to remove foods deemed to "pollute" the body, including alcohol, caffeine, refined sugar, and processed and fast food. The most extreme detox diets tend to be juice-based – that is, every meal is replaced with a vegetable and/or fruit juice for a few days at a time, usually during one week a month. At the other end of the scale, a detox diet might suggest high reliance on fruit and vegetable juices, supplemented with meals made up using white fish, chicken, and vegetables. Dairy, all carbohydrates except those in fruit and veg, fats, alcohol and caffeine are on the banned list. This kind of detox is usually more sustained, occurring over a predetermined, prolonged period of time, every day of the week.

Then, there are fasting diets – which are really just detox diets by another name. In these, the dieter can eat how he or she likes on, say, five days a week, but restrict calories to only 500 (for women) or 600 (for men) on two days a week.

The claims for most detox diets are that they will "reset" your digestive system – perhaps after a period of overindulgence, or as a way to even out consumption every week. The notion is that by giving your body a chance to flush out pollutants and impurities, it can work more efficiently and you will feel less sluggish.

The diets promise increased energy levels, weight loss, clearer skin, brighter eyes and, in women, a reduction in cellulite.

True or false gold?

Our bodies are naturally brilliant at resetting themselves. Although most of us inevitably have periods of the year when we overindulge – on holiday, at Christmas, over a birthday – is it really necessary, then, to have a digestive clean-out, or is this just a red herring?

Well, there is absolutely no scientific evidence to suggest that detox diets do in fact rid the body of toxins. The liver and digestive system are incredibly complex, well-designed functions in the magical machine of our physiology and they are supremely efficient at dealing with overindulgence without any external help.

While our waistbands may feel slightly tighter immediately after a holiday, with a few weeks of fairly normal eating and light to moderate exercise (or even just moving around more – walk up the stairs rather than taking the lift; get off the bus one stop earlier and walk the rest of the way), most people will easily shed any minor gain in weight.

Weight loss is one of the real drivers for a detox regimen. However, interestingly, while the scales may show that you have lost weight, actually all you've lost is fluid and stores of glycogen. Remember that when you remove carbohydrate from your diet, your body uses glycogen as its source of energy, depleting your stores. Lost glycogen can account for an apparent weight loss of around 2kg within a few days. True weight loss, though, is to do with losing body fat, not glycogen. Once you start eating normally again, glycogen stores are replenished, and the supposed weight loss turns into what appears to be weight gain.

Severely restrictive detox programmes are worst of all for making false promises. For weight loss to be sustainable, the body has to work with your goals, not against them. If you have a limited period of overindulgence, your body naturally raises your metabolism to cope with the extra calories. Initially, then, even though you might feel bigger, heavier, more sluggish, your body is doing a fine job all by itself of eventually restoring balance. If, though, after a period of overindulgence, you suddenly and drastically cut back on calories, your body goes into shock. It thinks there's famine and instead of raising your metabolism and burning more calories even at rest, it winds it back

– slowing it down to preserve what energy stores you have, including holding on to body fat.

The truth is that reducing our overall intake of caffeine, alcohol and processed foods is not harmful – we should all take note and cut back. However, remember that orthorexia is a psychological, obsessive condition. What starts out as a spring clean, by cutting back on substances in our food and drink that might be detrimental to our health, becomes increasingly more limiting – first processed foods, then carbohydrates, then fats... and so on. The list of "must-nots" becomes ever-longer turning spring-cleaning into a mania that is the sole focus of every waking minute.

Fundamentally, detox diets are not healthy. Many juice-based detoxes are very low in overall energy and while the intention may be to follow them only for a few days, they put the body under huge amounts of stress. Stress in itself generates toxicity in the body (prolonged raised cortisone levels disrupt all the body's systems, including its ability to remove environmental toxins) – so the net effect is potentially the very opposite of the intended effect. There are physical consequences. The quest is for weight loss, increased energy and clear skin, but the reality can be:

- Lack of energy

- Dizziness

- Nausea owing to low blood-sugar levels

- Stomach pain as a result of hunger pangs

- Food cravings, particularly sugar and carbohydrate, owing to the restrictive nature of the diet

- Nutritional deficiencies, especially if you follow the diet for a long period of time

How far is too far?

For many, a detox diet can be the start of a very unhealthy relationship with and attitude toward food. The notion that detox is a "cleansing process" legitimizes the idea that we should punish indulgence through a purge. This particular mentality can hook those individuals susceptible to, or already living with, orthorexia. The obsession takes over so much that eventually it's not genuine overindulgence that becomes the trigger for detox, but any small perceived nutritional misdemeanour. If they break just one, small food rule, they will follow a detox to make amends.

You can see how quickly a cycle of deprivation and punishment can take hold, even though it's not the food that causes the sense of impurity, but a psychology that is far less easy to fix.

IN SUMMARY

It would be impossible for me to cover every possible diet, its effects and rules and how those might be perceived by someone living with orthorexia – and even if I did so, by the time this book is published a whole new crop of pseudo-dietary advice and diet fads would be finding followers on the Internet. However, I hope that by covering the diets I most commonly see causing problems for those who come to see me in my clinic, I have shown how their promises are not all that they seem – that there is much false gold in the world of nutrition, and that the hallmarks of that false gold are common to whatever dietary fads might be around now or in the future.

Lack of genuine nutritional expertise in so many of those who promote, through blogs, websites, articles and books, a particular diet in the name of health and well-being is, in fact, perpetuating dis-ease. When one approach to eating appears to have a positive effect on one individual at one particular time in their life, we do not have a scientific study – it is not evidence; it's just the happy outcome for one individual. And I champion that – everyone should find what works for them. However, one happy story doesn't necessarily apply to all. If you are someone who has got stuck, or you know someone whose quest for healthy eating appears to have turned into an obsession, or you know of someone who is struggling with their approach to nutrition, keep reading. In the next chapter we are going to look at some practical strategies on how to break free from the "food rules".

CHAPTER 3

ESCAPING ORTHOREXIA

In the previous chapter we explored how our understanding of healthy eating and the role of nutrients in our diet have become confused, tainted and even extreme. The level of confusion that abounds regarding what it means to adopt healthy eating principles seems to be directly related to the increase in accessibility of nutritional knowledge. Like so many topics that were once the preserve of authoritative books or conversations with genuine experts, nutrition has become a topic for all – with lots of information (and misinformation) accessible on the Internet night and day, seven days a week.

Over the last two decades, there has been an astronomical rise in the level of interest about nutrition and nutritional principles. Increasingly, we have realized that what we eat really does have a significant impact on our health. It also means that we all have an opinion –

garnered from snippets we pick up here and there – on what's good for us and what's not. I really welcome this debate – nutrition is my livelihood and I love that as a demographic we are so much more conscious about what we eat than even our parents' generation, and that we care enough to form opinions and want to get our nutrition (and that of our families) right. However, I don't advocate anyone presenting opinion as fact (on nutrition, on carpentry, on the impact of nuclear power on the environment). Whatever the topic, when advice or information is based on someone's personal opinion, experience or viewpoint, we need to know so that we can treat that information lightly, in the spirit that it should be intended. To be fair, I believe that many people who share their nutritional success stories on the Internet intend to do just that – share a personal story in the hope that it might provide hope for someone reading it. I don't think there's necessarily any intent to mislead – rather, it's an excited reaction to feeling well, cured or just plain elated with life. I think, though, sometimes unregulated, uncorroborated, unsubstantiated stories of personal success are dangerous when they are so readily accessible to impressionable Internet searchers, who are looking for answers.

It is highly likely that if someone becomes more mindful about their dietary intake, choosing fewer processed foods and cooking from scratch instead of heating things up from a packet, the result will be an improved sense of well-being. In most cases, I believe, it's not the removal of a particular nutrient or food group that has effected change, but the other dietary changes that removing that food group forces. For a person struggling with orthorexia, this logic doesn't hold any appeal: in the quest for pure health an orthorexic will remove all foods deemed unhealthy – even when there is no scientific proof that the banned foods are harmful to the body. The real worry about this is that often removing everything can create more problems than its solves, both mentally and physically – after all, this isn't how the human body was intended to survive.

CASE STUDY

EXPERTISE MATTERS

A woman in her 20s who had recently been diagnosed with Crohn's disease (a type of inflammatory bowel disease) came to see me. She was on steroid medication, but her symptoms were still very severe. The ongoing symptoms and the side-effects of the medication were damaging her confidence. Desperate to find something (anything) that would help, several weeks before coming to me, she had been to see a "nutritional coach", whom she had found online. The coach ran some allergy tests that concluded that her symptoms were not related to Crohn's disease, but that instead she was allergic to wheat, gluten, dairy and sugar. On the advice of the coach, the woman modified her diet to accommodate the allergies the coach had apparently identified in her. Four weeks later, instead of an improvement in her symptoms, she was feeling worse. By the time she came to me, she was exhausted and emotional.

The standard clinical treatment for active Crohn's disease is steroids and then something called a "Few Foods Diet". Sufferers of the disease are given the principles of the diet under the instruction of a registered clinical dietitian, who follows and guides their progress closely. On the Few Foods Diet, the sufferer removes the food groups that the gastro-intestinal system can find difficult to break down and absorb, particularly when it is inflamed. He or she must follow the diet only for short periods of time, then one by one reintroduce each food, at a rate of one every 24 hours. If the patient suffers an adverse reaction, that particular food is removed again. Over several weeks, he or she will then be able to build up a relatively normal diet containing foods that don't cause a reaction. With my help, after three months following the Few Foods Diet, my client was able to reintroduce dairy, gluten, wheat and sugar, and she felt better than she'd felt in a long while.

The point of this story is to highlight that the Internet, wonderful as it is, does not regulate who posts what, or who claims to be an expert in any particular field. It means that anyone who is desperate for an answer to a particular problem is susceptible to misinformation and even, when we're talking about health and well-being, misdiagnosis. As we sift through information online, it's becoming increasingly hard to assess what comes from a genuine "expert" and what comes from a well-meaning storyteller – and once you start to promote what one, perhaps unqualified, person is telling you above what your body's telling you, you hit a danger zone.

THE OTHER CULPRITS

Of course, it's not just the Internet and accessibility of misinformation that's to blame for why we are where we are with modern attitudes to nutrition. I think there are other reasons our approach to our diet has become skewed:

- Food is more readily available – most of us live in places where we can buy groceries or order take-aways late into the night, if not all night, every day of the week.

- We crave convenience – as our lives have become busier, we have found ourselves using more ready-to-eat products rather than cooking from scratch.

- We have far greater access to good information, too – and we hear every new discovery as it happens. The result is that we don't know what to believe and what not to believe.

- We are under far greater pressure to be successful and perfect in every way – and we allow that need for perfection to permeate all aspects of our lives.

But, returning to a state of palaeolithic eating isn't the answer either – after all, humankind has adapted to become far more highly skilled and intelligent over thousands of years of evolution than it was at the dawn of human existence. If our prehistoric ancestors had it right, evolution wouldn't be as we see it today.

Perhaps, then, there's something in-between. When you speak to the older generation, they often talk about how life was "simpler" when they were young. Indeed, studies and statistics show time and again that we were healthier during the World Wars. The main reason for this is rationing, or to give it a rather less alarming term, moderation. During the wars, out of necessity, we were forced to eat healthy portion sizes of nutrient-rich, home-prepared foods. Is this the answer to the problem of orthorexia – to try to re-educate a highly demanding, self-critical generation that in fact perfection lies in something as boring and uninspiring as being moderate?

WHAT IS MODERATION?

I am often reluctant to spell out what we mean by terms such as low, moderate and high, mostly because our individual body composition and exercise levels change what these things mean for different people. Nonetheless, as a starting point it can be helpful to know what moderate is in light of broad categories of health and lifestyle. The most important thing to take from these broad examples is that regardless of your genetics or lifestyle, no food is demonized and you eat from all the food groups. Fundamentally, there is balance.

Moderate means:

- For the predominantly sedentary individual who may want to lose or maintain weight, sticking to three meals a day, all containing a balance of carbohydrate, protein, vegetables or salad and some essential fats daily; with one or two snacks of mainly fruit or low-fat dairy and keeping foods high in fat and sugar or meals out to no more than once or twice a week.

- For the moderately active individual trying to maintain weight, sticking to three meals, all containing a balance of carbohydrate, protein, vegetables or salad and some essential fats daily; with two or three snacks of small portions of nuts, fruit and dairy or small portions of wholegrain carbohydrates such as oatcakes with cheese, and keeping foods high in fat and sugar or meals out to no more than two to three times a week.

- For those who are very active or who do not put weight on quickly and may even need to gain weight, sticking to three meals, all containing a balance of carbohydrate, protein, vegetables or salad and some essential fats daily; with two or three snacks of combinations of two or more food groups, such as toast with mashed avocado or a bowl of cereal or fruit, yogurt and toasted seeds; occasionally eating meals out; and keeping quantities of foods high in fat and sugar small – such as, a few squares of chocolate or a piece of cake or a couple of biscuits once a day.

The trouble is, we don't like the word "moderate" or any of its derivatives. It doesn't have the positive, sexy, go-getter connotations that epitomizes success for a high-achieving generation. Whenever I use the term "moderation" in clinic, workshops or presentations, I can see people screw up their noses.

Moderation is hard – it is about balance. Rationing (albeit the result of horrific circumstances) forced portion control. There were no decisions to make about when enough was enough, it just was. Furthermore, meals and snacks had to be cooked from scratch because there was no processed food.

However, moderation also means being moderate in our attitudes. While I am all for cooking from scratch, I don't beat myself up if I have to use a jar of pasta sauce now and again; but I wouldn't be happy if I were eating mostly processed food all the time. We do know that if your diet is made up of predominantly non-nutrient-dense choices such as fizzy drinks, white bread and processed meat, you are more likely to become overweight, and suffer the poor health associated with being so.

HEALTHY PLATEFULS – THE DIETITIAN'S VIEW

So how do we get the balance right? How do we move out of the mindset that answers lie in extremes, achieve moderation and feel it's a positive thing. How do we make moderation an appealing way to look at nutrition to the extent that it becomes more appealing than being locked in the grip of an eating disorder?

Take the long view

First, think of the freedom and sense of relief that comes from releasing a sense of panic that every day must be perfect. Instead, consider a more long-term strategy. Relieving pressure and immediacy is a way to feel more instantly positive about yourself and life.

A healthy diet is actually about the nutritional balance we achieve over a period of time; it is not specific to each day. While you may aim to hit a target of eating five to eight fruits or vegetables a day, some days you may only manage just one or two, while on other days you may eat nine or ten. Over the course of a month or even a year, in general your nutritional choices – as long as they are generally consciously healthy ones – will balance out the maths.

In the same way, on some days work, study or family life may railroad all your best intentions and what in the morning you thought would be a hand-prepared supper, cooked from scratch, by 6pm is a readymade pizza thrown into the oven. It's not ideal, but if it happens only occasionally, you aren't unhealthy – you're human. It's all about the overall trend.

Try to look at the balance you achieve over a period of seven to ten days during a normal working week (or over a month if you have a more indulgent holiday), as this gives you a much more realistic view of your nutritional intake. If over one ten-day period it seems your intake of sugar or saturated fat has been a bit overindulgent – just be more mindful over the next ten-day period. Allow moderation to be liberating.

Personalize it

Second, think about you. Yes, you – your unique, brilliant, individual self. For some, a hearty bowl of porridge with toasted seeds is the perfect start to the day, maintaining energy levels and keeping us satisfied all the way through to lunch. However, for others, a few hours after a bowl of porridge, the hunger pangs start. Instead, only wholegrain toast with peanut butter will do the job. Both options are good – each provides a healthy mix of wholegrain carbohydrate, essential fats and protein – the difference is personal choice. In the same way, some days you may not feel like eating either of these options and only toast and marmalade or a coffee and croissant will do. Okay, that won't make for the healthiest day of your life – but does it matter once in a while? No, of course not. Let your choices reflect what your unique body is telling you.

Think of food as friend

Food is more than just energy; food has a huge role to play in our lives: it develops sociability, it is comforting and sustaining, and it can significantly influence your mood – just like a good friend. Scientific studies show that when food becomes an issue or causes anxiety, the result is low mood and, in severe cases, depression.

Categorizing foods as "good" or "bad" influences how we respond to them, even before they've touched our lips. So, for example, if I believed that croissants were "bad" for me, but I ate one anyway, my response would be guilt, anxiety and self-deprecation. If the food is bad, then I am bad for eating it.

Furthermore, if we label a food as bad, we're likely to deprive ourselves of it. Then what happens? For most people that deprivation leads to total preoccupation – I can't have it, so I want it, but I mustn't have it, what will happen if I do have it, I'll feel bad about it, so I mustn't... And so the self-talk goes on. In this way deprivation leads to obsessional behaviour – characteristic of orthorexia.

In my mind all foods are friends – but like friends, there are some you want to spend more time with than others.

THE PERILS OF A BEST FRIEND

I've used the analogy that we should treat food as our friend, but what happens with we concentrate on one friend and believe that friend is the answer to all our problems. The chances are, the burden on the friendship is too great – you might get on each other's nerves, or even get to the point when you can't bear to be in each other's company. Here, we're back to moderation. While characteristically orthorexia leads to food rules that result in deprivation, there are also occasions when the rules place magical powers on one particular nutrient or foodstuff. Superfoods, that is foods with particularly special nutritional powers, commonly cited include coconut oil, goji berries and kale or green juice. But just as no single food causes cause ill health, nor does any single food really have superpowers. I think there are key ingredients that it's good to use because they contain beneficial nutrients. The truth is, though, that in a balanced, moderate diet, you should get all the key nutrients you need for good health. Reliance on a single super-friend is just as much of a red herring as banishing a friend you think is harming you.

Build a healthy plateful

Understanding what constitutes a properly healthy plate of food can help those in recovery from eating disorders, including orthorexia. The following suggestions are merely to demonstrate what a healthy, balanced meal or snack might look like – they are by no means rules! They are a guide to help you produce balanced meals and snacks.

However, don't expect too much too soon – remember that with orthorexia the established rules are deeply embedded with so much hingeing on them in terms of self-esteem, often over and above body image. Make small changes aiming for a properly healthy plate of food eventually. A healthy diet is the destination you're aiming for, but the road there may be a long one. In many situations, as well as changing food habits, it will take significant and ongoing psychological support to deal with the underlying issues that trigger orthorexia and are often not related to food at all.

I'm a big fan of splitting a plate into three, which provides a simple guideline for how to balance out a meal. Aim to make one third of the food on your plate nutrient-dense carbohydrates (for example, oats, sweet or white potatoes), bread (ideally wholegrain, but not necessarily – opt for a loaf you slice yourself, rather than processed sliced bread, though), or rice or pasta (again, ideally wholegrain for its fibre, but not essentially). Another third of the portion can be protein in the form of fish, meat, poultry, beans or pulses, tofu, or eggs. For the final third, have vegetables or salad foods.

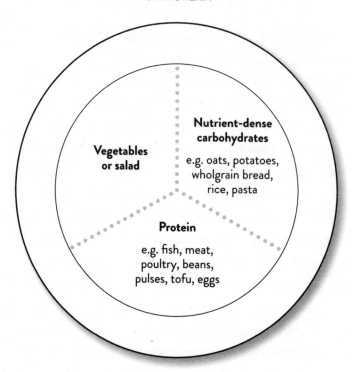

Try to include foods that provide you with essential fats (nuts, seeds and avocados, for example) and try to include dairy – three servings a day will provide you with your body's daily calcium requirements. A serving is, for example, one third of a pint of whole milk, a matchbox-sized portion of cheese, or 150g yogurt.

And don't forget that these are guidelines, not rules: if you exercise three or four times a week, you might need more of any particular nutrient; if you exercise five or six times, still more. Part of the road to recovery is learning to listen to and trust your body, and responding accordingly.

Finally, don't forget the unrestrained eating theory – nothing is off limits in moderation. So, yes, I've just described a healthy, moderate way to fill your plate, but that doesn't mean you can't have a chocolate bar every now and then, just don't have two or three every day. And try not to view these foods as a treat – just view them as a minor part of a healthy, balanced diet.

Listen to your body

One of the biggest barriers for those recovering from orthorexia is trusting that if they relax the rules a little, they will know when to stop. In other words, if chips are on the banned list, they worry that one chip will lead to a whole portion, which will lead to a whole portion every week, then every day and so on.

The body is an amazing machine – the most intricate and finely tuned you will ever discover. Typically, when it's been deprived of something – especially if that something has deprived it of energy – it will crave it, indulge in it and use it to replenish stores, just in case it ever becomes starved of energy again. However, once it realizes that there is balance – that eating is regular and the nutritional value of each meal is sufficient for good health, its alert system downgrades from red to amber and then eventually to green – the threat has passed and normal metabolism and appetite are restored. Your body learns to re-regulate.

Remember that the driving force for orthorexia is not usually to lose weight, it is purity. Nonetheless, the result is deprivation. It may not be that you've deprived your body of energy; it may be a particular nutrient or particular set of nutrients that your body desperately needs. Once stocks are replenished and the body learns to relax again, any cravings will pass.

We're all born with this innate ability – if you've ever spent any time with small children, you'll know that they are brilliant at demanding very specific foods when something is lacking. They instinctively know what they want to eat and when. I know that when they were little, my own daughters would go through phases of eating just the carbohydrate element of their meals; then other weeks they seemed only to be eating the dairy or protein. While this was frustrating, I never stressed about it too much, as I knew that they were tuning in to what their bodies wanted and actually, when looking at the bigger picture, they were getting a balanced diet.

MEAL IDEAS

As I've said, this book isn't a nutritional handbook intended to offer a new set of rules to live by. Nonetheless, I appreciate that it can be helpful to see the theory put into practice. So, as a guide here are some food ideas to get you started on the path to wellness.

BREAKFASTS

- Wholegrain or sourdough toast with nut butter and a piece of fruit
- Porridge made with milk and topped with toasted seeds and homemade fruit compote
- Bowl of muesli, topped with Greek yogurt and fresh fruit
- Wholegrain or sourdough toast with scrambled or poached eggs, served with ½ avocado
- Homemade pancakes with frozen berries, honey and Greek yogurt
- Bowl of Greek yogurt with fruit and honey, followed by a croissant

MEAL IDEAS FOR LUNCH AND SUPPER

- Chicken or tofu stir-fry with rice
- Chickpea and vegetable curry with a pitta

- Coconut and lentil soup with sweet-potato bites
- Jacket potato with hummus and avocado salad
- Roasted vegetable and feta bruschetta
- Vegetable and cheese frittata with a pitta and a salad
- Sausage casserole with fresh bread
- Pasta with tomato, olive and cannellini bean sauce
- Fish pie with steamed mixed vegetables
- Baked salmon with jacket wedges, peas and a squeeze of lemon

SNACKS
- Seeded oatcakes with hummus or nut butter
- Greek yogurt, fruit and honey
- Toasted tea cake or fruit scone with butter
- Slice of homemade banana bread
- Bowl of cereal with milk
- Fruit and yogurt smoothie
- Glass of milk and a couple of large squares of chocolate
- Dried fruit and nuts
- Toast

CARING FOR YOUR MIND

While understanding what to eat is one aspect of recovering from orthorexia, the biggest challenge is freeing yourself from the anxieties that you have developed relating to food and its apparent ability to make your body pure or impure, as the case may be.

FEELING WORSE TO FEEL BETTER

When you first embark upon your recovery journey, perhaps taking additional support in the form of a counsellor or psychologist who can help you with underlying emotional concerns, and help you to build your emotional resilience, you may at first feel worse (that is, more emotionally unstable, or more anxious) – this is perfectly normal. The most important thing is that you understand the process and ask for help to get you through it – and that you don't give up. Taking the first step to recovery is the hardest: try to keep moving forward, leaning on those you love and trust to help and support you.

The underlying driver for orthorexia is trying to establish purity. But what makes a person feel impure in the first place? In most of the cases I have seen, the sufferers don't feel good enough. That feeling of inadequacy rarely stems from body image, but is an irrational thought or belief that stems from the experiences of life – sometimes one particular experience, and sometimes just ongoing negativity.

In Chapter 1, I gave a case study about a teenager who tried to control her diet as a means to deal with her acne and in doing so developed orthorexia. Most teenagers are self conscious – it goes with the territory, but what makes one teenager shrug his or her shoulders at the spots, rationalize that they will pass and so just get on with life, while another chronically feels so inadequate that he or she needs to act on this through extreme methods that develop into a significant eating disorder? I'm not a psychologist but I do know that in this case, the teenager had a pretty tricky home life. Her brother was disabled and her mother wasn't well. While her father did the best for them all, my client always felt like third best – inevitably, her dad's focus needed to be her brother and her mother. She felt that she was never good enough to get her father's full attention.

In fact, the situation itself was her own interpretation of the reality of what was happening. Nonetheless, this is how she perceived it and her illness was not really a result of whether or not she could get rid of the acne, but a way in which to punish herself for not being good enough. Her acne wasn't actually that bad at all, but it became a physical representation of her unhappiness; and the orthorexia gave her a physical outlet, a punishment for her inadequacies. Her acne was a physical trigger for an unhealthy relationship with food – but neither the acne nor the eating disorder were really the root of the problem. Interestingly, when she met someone who made her feel accepted and provided her with the care and attention she craved, she saw her life in a far more rational light. Her relationship enabled her to step back, assess what was going on, and take positive steps to get better.

This example demonstrates how orthorexia is just an outlet. It can take hold, but it's not really the heart of the problem; controlling food validates existence – "While I can follow the rules, I am worth something." That's why it's so hard to overcome.

One of the things I say to all my clients is that in order to get better, they need to get comfortable with the uncomfortable. Challenging eating behaviours to include some of your "forbidden foods" is hugely stressful for someone with an eating disorder. Anxiety is completely normal – the key is for the sufferer to allow him- or herself to experience their feelings and just keep reassuring themselves that nothing awful is going to happen when a rule gets broken. At the start, eating "impure" foods needs to become a rule in itself, something that is a deliberate practice. When a sufferer starts to see that eating a forbidden food doesn't have catastrophic consequences, slowly and with small steps, he or she can build the confidence to re-establish normal eating patterns.

This takes time, so I usually set goals. For example, for someone who has removed all gluten for no medical reason, I would first suggest swapping one gluten-free choice for a standard option. So, the sufferer might have regular toast for breakfast, rather than toast made with gluten-free bread. Once he or she can do this without a sense of deep anxiety and can articulate that he or she accepts that there have been no dreadful consequences, I move onto the next challenge (a bowl of regular pasta for supper once a week, for example). The process can take months and even years, but a slow recovery is, in my view, more likely to be a sustainable recovery.

WHAT ABOUT EXERCISE?

So far we have concentrated on how an individual with orthorexia fixates on food rules, but as I said at the start of the book, increasingly orthorexia includes "clean living" as well as "clean eating" and this means looking at the role of exercise, too. There has been a recent surge in a concept of "fitspo", that is fitness inspiration. It has become the hashtag for anyone that wants to be associated with fitness and healthy living and definitely plays into the hands of the orthorexic.

If you type #fitspo into Instagram, it comes up with 39,444,157 posts (2017); similarly, #fitsporation has 1,170,254 posts (2017). Click on any of these and you are inundated with individuals taking selfies of themselves in gym kit, showing off toned abdominals, working out in the gym, or presenting a picture of what they deem the perfect fuel for their workout. Rather like "clean eating", fitspo masquerades as something that can only be good for you – but there is potential harm in such a "perfect" body image. While a fitness guru is proud of his or her washboard stomach and bulging biceps, they're unaware what a negative influence this has on so many.

In my role as a dietitian I work with elite athletes in many different sports. I am a huge advocate of the fitness industry – but not when it presents false information or promise; just as I believe in educating people about good nutrition, but not at the expense of health. Do images of "perfect" bodies encourage a healthy lifestyle, or do they lead to obsessive pursuit of perfection that in susceptible individuals may cause more harm than good?

While it's not central to a diagnosis of orthorexia to focus on a perfect body, like those with other eating disorders orthorexics have a constant negative internal narrative – they see themselves in a negative light or deem themselves "not good enough", including sometimes in terms of their physical appearance. Fitspo feeds the negative cycle, validating feelings of inadequacy and therefore fuelling the drive for more control in the pursuit of physical purity and perfection – through food and exercise.

A piece of research published in the journal *Appetite* in February 2017 concluded that sports study students demonstrated an increased tendency toward orthorexia compared with those doing business studies. Interestingly perhaps (especially given that anorexia and bulimia tend to occur more frequently in women), the trend was actually more pronounced in male sports science students than in female. The researchers hypothesized on the impact of this trend for future populations, given that most of the students intended to go on to coach other, impressionable sportsmen and -women. If a cohort of sports coaches has fixed ideas relating to nutrition, body image, and exercise, based on each coach's own eating disorder, would this become perpetuated throughout the training and coaching pathway? They concluded that probably yes, it would.

So, what came first? Is it that a move toward a healthier way of life begins with exercise and extends to diet, and then a pursuit of clean eating and eventually perhaps orthorexia; or is it that when nutritional changes don't fulfil the need to be clean and pure (they never will because they aren't actually the answer to the orthorexic's problems), a sufferer takes a new tack and adds exercise to the rules by which to live? Does it really matter? Either way, food and exercise become obsessional, all-consuming and debilitating.

EXERCISE IN OTHER EATING DISORDERS

Exercise addiction is characteristic of all eating disorders, not just orthorexia. In anorexia and bulimia, sufferers use exercise to assist their weight control and "reset" the counters when they feel they have fallen off the wagon in some way. Many anorexics talk about feeling as though they are unworthy or undeserving of food unless they exercise. While this demonstrates a desire to eat, the focus is on exercise as the trigger for eating. The amount of exercise that becomes the trigger point for being worthy often gets more and more difficult to achieve, especially as the sufferer gets weaker – creating a never-ending cycle of malnourishment, weight loss and weakness. The truth of it is that the anorexic individual does not feel worthy of allowing him- or herself to eat – full stop.

Bound up in all that is a diminished sense of self-worth. Exercise becomes an additional way to purge feelings of inadequacy – because someone with an eating disorder never feels good enough, he or she keeps pushing the body to the edge of its limits in order to prove he or she can do it. Only enough is never enough and the cycle never ends.

Just as dietary changes may start off perfectly innocently, in orthorexia what begins as a healthy attempt to exercise two or three times a week, gradually becomes more punishing. Some of my clients come to me when they are exercising two or three times a day. If a social event interferes with the exercise or diet regime, the social event is cancelled. Going on holiday and missing exercise classes or scheduled runs will cause a sense of panic. If he or she doesn't meet their workout commitments, they believe that disaster will ensue.

It is really important to stress here that just as with food, while a health-conscious person will care about their body and health, an individual with orthorexia becomes completely fixated and obsessed to the point of ill health. When exercise becomes something they "have" to do rather than "want" to do, it is often a sign that there is a much bigger problem.

Breaking this destructive cycle takes time and patience. Levels of anxiety associated with reducing or even stopping exercise, are heightened, causing huge amounts of distress. Just as with reintroducing foods, the steps to overcoming the mindset need to be tiny and methodical – until finally the sufferer reaches a point of acceptance that the world will keep turning, even if they miss a run. In other words, escaping orthorexia needs (you guessed it) moderation.

OLD HABITS DIE HARD

I recently spoke to two clients on separate occasions. Both are in the recovery stages of their orthorexia, having become aware that their nutritional practices (in both cases restricting carbohydrates and dairy) have adversely affected their health and well-being. While they are both committed to returning to a state of well-being and balance, they both admitted that their old behaviours – the ones that kept them locked in the cycle of orthorexia – and internal negative dialogues were very hard to let go. Both women are fully aware of the benefits that certain carbohydrates and dairy foods bring to their long-term health, but when they eat these foods, they still feel a sense of guilt and failure.

I am extremely proud of both of them, because even though the guilt still surfaces, they have each started to take charge of their own futures. They are no longer slaves to their disease, but their roads to recovery will be long and fraught with difficulties and doubts and yet they are sticking with it. I am delighted that they have both come to me to help them put right their nutritional choices; and both are getting psychological help, too.

A HEALTHY ATTITUDE TO SELF

So, we've established that the root of the problem, the reason for needing to find control through restricting food or undertaking a punishing exercise regime lies a lot deeper than simply what's on a plate or how many times you make it to the gym in a day. It lies with the sense of self. Orthorexia is a mental illness – you can't just snap out of it, because there needs to be a shift in attitude not just toward food or exercise, but toward our own sense of identity. While education about food is essential, it's really only treating the symptom. To recover from any disease, we need to treat the underlying cause.

FINDING MODERATION BEYOND FOOD

You'll know by now that one of my favourite words is "moderation". However, this doesn't apply just to food. A healthy attitude to the self means accepting and even seeking out moderation in all things in life, from relationships to work to family. Let's go back to our friendship analogy (see page 126). Extremes of friendship are often incredibly unhealthy – whether overly intense or hand-wavingly dismissive, a friendship that has no middle ground, no come-and-go can be stressful and even damaging. On the other hand, friendships that have a gentle, unjudgemental easiness often work best – these are friendships that enjoy moderation. It doesn't mean they are necessarily any less loyal or loving than an intense friendship, just that they come with an unconditional familiarity and trust that makes them easy and healthy. The same principles can be applied to attitudes to work. A job that pushes you to your limits to the point of feeling you have to prove yourself or push yourself further or risk a sense of inadequacy isn't as healthy as the job that comes with moderation – a time for work and a time for play.

So, even though most of this book has focused on understanding and breaking down unnecessary food rules, in fact recovery from orthorexia starts with our relationship with the self; and in my view it's the most important part. Being able to demonstrate self-compassion rather than constantly trying to run away, squash or control feelings of discomfort, is a fundamental to the recovery process.

If orthorexia is the pursuit of physical purity and perfection, what do purity and perfection actually look like? The truth is that what I think makes me pure and perfect is likely to be quite different from what you want to achieve for your own purity. In which case, our journey toward self-compassion is very individual. What is perfect for one person is not the same for another.

Nonetheless, there are certain parameters that definitely do apply to us all. The first and most significant is that you cannot achieve happiness or self-acceptance through the food that you eat. When you read bold statements online about how if you eat a certain way you will find self-fulfilment because you'll cure illness, improve your skin tone, or have more energy – it's not true. There may be physical benefits to eating a well-balanced diet (yes, it will show in your skin, hair and nails), but individual food fads that require you to remove a food group from your diet will not lead to physical perfection and they definitely won't make you feel happy. Not really happy, not deep-down, long-lasting, self-loving, believe-in-yourself happy.

For that you need to learn to be at ease with yourself and that means finding out what has triggered your lack of self-worth. For some it might be a negative childhood experience – such as bullying or a difficult relationship with a parent – that remains deep-rooted and unaddressed for many years, only to emerge as an eating disorder. For others, it may be a relationship breakdown or the sudden, unexpected loss of a loved one that manifests as some kind of failure. Once the mindset of lack of worth has taken hold, it can seem the whole world is affirming that place of self-loathing:

"I wasn't good enough for that role and that's why they let me go"

or, "I didn't try hard enough to please my partner; they deserve better; no wonder he/she doesn't want to be with me any more."

In counselling, therapists will work with individuals to understand their story and then help them to unpick the negative narrative, exchanging it for a far more positive internal dialogue. Learning self-compassion is one of the key features of recovery from an eating disorder such as orthorexia.

Finding self-compassion

The word compassion means to "suffer with" – to show compassion for others means to feel another person's pain, to empathise with them and to show warmth and care with the aim of alleviating their suffering. Being compassionate toward someone else means offering them understanding, kindness and, if necessary, forgiveness – or showing them the way to forgive themselves. When you feel compassion for another person, you show that you appreciate that suffering, failure and imperfection are all part of life.

Self-compassion means that you behave in the same way toward yourself. If you are having a difficult time, fail at a task or notice something you don't like about yourself, instead of trying to ignore this pain and discomfort or berate yourself for it, you stop to tell yourself, "This is really difficult right now, how can I comfort and care for myself in this moment?"

You do this instead of judging and criticizing yourself for your perceived inadequacies or shortcomings. One of the most important things about showing self-compassion is that you honour and accept what it means to be human and imperfect. Life doesn't always go the way we want – each of us will experience loss and sadness in our lifetime; sometimes we may seem to fail and other times reach our limitations, but it's important to remember that those are the normal experiences of a normal life, and we all have to cope with rocky roads from time to time. In addition, most of us go through periods (some shorter than others) of believing we aren't worthy of our own love, let alone the love of someone else. But why? What is it that we are expecting of life and ourselves? Recovering from orthorexia requires letting go of the notion that we have to be perfect, stopping running away from our emotions, accepting them even when they are painful and opening the door to self-compassion.

I believe that recovering from orthorexia not only needs work with a dietitian, but also with a therapist, psychologist or psychotherapist. Alongside that professional psychological help, I encourage my clients to use some simple exercises to support their mental well-being as they begin their road to recovery, with the destination being a restored sense of well-being in the physical, mental and emotional self. While this might manifest in eating healthy, balanced meals, and relaxing food rules, the real journey's end occurs when my clients can demonstrate self-compassion.

Step 1: Build your road

I use the road analogy with my clients as a means to start their self-help programme in the following way.

Your destination is your full recovery, but to get there you have to build a road with motivational signposting and milestones that encourage you to keep going and show you are making progress. What motivates you to keep going? Draw a main road on a large piece of paper (allow the road to twist and turn so that you can give yourself lots of space). Along this main road, document situations or people that keep you motivated to stay on the road – these will be the situations you enjoy and the people you love most who help you want to get well. For example, you might draw an image of a cinema to represent being able to go out to the cinema and enjoy the company of your friends. You might draw a cupcake to represent the pleasure you derive from baking with your children; or the flag of a foreign country where you want to be able to go on holiday. Try turning those motivational situations into specific goals. So, as orthorexia usually forces deprivation of certain food groups, perhaps you would add milestones to represent related food goals. Perhaps you add a milestone at the cinema that represents your ability to eat popcorn; or at the baking image to eat one of the cakes you've made; or at the holiday image, to eat a croissant on your holiday in France.

In addition, try adding further milestones that might not be related to the motivators on your journey at all. For example, you might add a milestone at which you'll have a dessert, another for going out for a meal, another for reducing your exercise regime by one session, and another for doing something positive for yourself that demonstrates self-compassion – perhaps treating yourself to a long soak in a bubble bath, rather than going for a run. Or, perhaps going for a run, rather than staying in the office until after everyone else has gone home.

Every journey has alternative routes, detours that can take you off track – it is important to recognize these unwelcome paths so that you can stop at the junction and choose to stay on course. Draw little side routes with dead ends that draw you off your main road. Label these with signposts for the red herrings or setbacks that you know you'll have to watch out for. Don't worry if you can't think of these as you begin – you can add them in as they crop up to remind yourself not to be caught out by them later in your journey. Examples might be physical discomfort (feeling bloated because you've reintroduced something you've banned yourself from eating), guilt, anxiety, fear, anger, resentment and what others will think of you.

Now you have built your road, keep it with you or take a picture on your phone so that you can refer to it as often as you need. Either way, store the original. As you identify more trigger points or goals, add them to the road. What you'll end up with is a landscape to guide your recovery, reminding you what to aim for, and what to avoid.

Step 2: Practise acceptance

Think about yourself as a whole – all parts of you. Individuals with orthorexia tend only to want to focus on those traits they think others accept such as: being caring, fun, happy, clever, and so on. They don't like people to see the aspects of their personality that they feel represent negative character traits, such as being prone to anger or jealously, or being lazy or selfish.

However, it is important to remember that we all are made up of many character traits that work together to create our whole. We need to accept all these traits in ourselves in order to be able to continue down our road to recovery. So while you may not want to admit that you would rather watch TV one night than go for a run, remind yourself that a healthy body needs downtime and if your body is telling you it's tired, you need to rest. If you are quick to fly off the handle, remind yourself that your emotional response to situations is a sign that you feel deeply, passionately about things – a character trait to be celebrated.

Step 3: Practise positive self-talk

Those suffering from orthorexia struggle with seeing past their pervading negative self-image and the negative, critical self-chatter that goes on in their heads. For this reason, I often ask my clients to practise the following exercise that aims to realign the negative self-talk into something more positive.

First, write two lists relating to yourself – one list should comprise the things you like about yourself, and the other the things you don't like about yourself (in my experience, the list of negatives is likely to be longer than the list of positives). Put the lists aside, then identify three people in your life who are important to you. On a new piece of paper, write down what makes each of these people important to you – come up with at least three character traits and be specific. Think about the traits that you love about each person.

When you're satisfied you've covered their positives, consider how those character traits are reflected in each person's relationship with you. The aim is to demonstrate that the positive traits you see in others exist because those people feel positively about you and respond to you in a positive way.

For example, you may write the following list relating to your best friend:

Caring, accepting, makes me laugh.

Now look back at your list of negatives. Let's say that you've written that you are "unworthy, unkind, bad company". Challenge that negative narrative.

"If I were really unworthy, would <best friend> demonstrate their caring side toward me?"

"If my flaws were really as bad as I consider them to be and if I were really that unkind, would <best friend> really be as accepting of me?"

"If I were really that bad company, would <best friend> really want to spend time with me, having fun and making me laugh?"

Think about each of your negative attributes in light of the positive attributes you see in your friend. One by one, pick them off.

Step 4: Separate your thoughts

While you can use the positive self-talk exercise to turn specific comments in your negative inner dialogue into positive ones, or to remove them from your thoughts altogether, it's important also to understand that those negative thoughts are not your own, true inner voice, but the voice of your illness. I encourage my clients to listen intently to a snapshot of the dialogue that drives their orthorexia and to write it down as it happens. So, a conversation with your inner orthorexic critic may go something like this:

You: "I really miss hanging out with my friends and being able to eat pizza with them."

Inner critic: "Why do you want to hang out with them? Can they not see how much harm they are doing to themselves by encouraging each other to eat pizza? Your approach is better than that."

You: "I guess, but they always seem to have so much fun, chatting and laughing, I would like to have some fun, too."

Inner critic: "We are having fun – look at all these lovely gluten-free goodies we are going to make; and anyway, social fun is overrated. It's meaningless. What we're doing is keeping you pure and healthy – a much better use of your time."

Through this exercise you can start to clearly articulate what's going on in your head. Seen on paper, you can separate your own, rational voice from the voice that drives your orthorexic thought processes and steers you off the course of reason. You can see what you actually want versus the behaviours that represent the illness rather than you, the person. Learning to understand that these negative thoughts are a part of you, but also separate from you, you can start to see how they can make you unhappy and uncomfortable. Separating yourself from them in this way enables you to accept that they happen, but that you have control over whether or not you listen to them and work with them. You can learn to distance yourself from them, and even ignore and defy them.

Recovery is a personal journey with no right or wrong route. You will need to work out what approaches work best for you. However, in my experience the best outcomes occur when, first, you are ready to evoke change. And, second, you have a good support network of family and friends. Finally, please find a counsellor and a registered dietitian and work with both of them simultaneously – tackling both the cause and the symptom is the recipe for long-lasting recovery.

CASE STUDY

ANSWERS WITHIN, NOT WITHOUT

When I'm working with orthorexic patients, my main role as a dietitian is to offer the rational voice, so powerfully shouted down by the inner critic, a chance to come forward. By articulating what's already there, but drowned out, I can help my clients to hear the rational voice more clearly. The following is an example of a conversation I have had with one of my orthorexia clients. She had been following a plant-based diet but also restricted sugar and gluten. She admitted that when she started out, she did so because she was following a well-known food blogger and felt that the blogger's approach would help her to feel better about herself; help her to feel pure.

One of the first admissions she made as she began her recovery was that she desperately missed dairy foods – but that the pull to remove them in the name of purity was too strong for her to overcome.

Client: "It's just like everywhere I go, everything I see makes me feel confused about what to do, what to eat etc. Lots of stuff about how dairy is really bad, like this article? What do you think?"

Me: "I think that you can find a reason not to eat food if you look hard enough – this is part of your orthorexia, but the question I would ask you is what do you want to eat? I read articles like this and think yes fair point, but then before I decide to act on it, or incorporate it into my practice I also ask myself first, is it a credible article? And, second, I like cheese and it's good for my bones and teeth and so do I really want to give it up?"

Client: "Yeah, I suppose; I like cheese as well! There's probably not a single food that at least one person thinks should be avoided... There's just so much pressure to be a vegan... the majority of people I know with eating issues, such as orthorexia, are vegan."

▷

The client was looking for my approval. She doesn't feel worthy enough to have her own opinion about how she should eat to nourish her body; or to trust her own instincts about whether or not she should eat dairy. Instead she has been following a popular food fad she has found on the Internet, because of the writer's association with being a "clean eater" – and slender and beautiful, to boot. My role is to help the client find the inner resilience to trust her instincts, to disentangle herself from the nutrition myths that she has learned over the previous years and to think about what she wants to eat or to avoid and why, and to balance her nutritional intake accordingly – even if that means helping her through the process of reintroducing cheese and dairy.

CHAPTER 4

EMBRACING THE FUTURE

· ·

When I've worked with clients who have made the decision to move forward out of the grip of orthorexia, the emotional release feels monumental and overwhelming. I reassure them that it takes a lot of strength to appreciate that the path you have previously chosen as a means of improving yourself has actually had the opposite effect on your well-being. Making the decision to undo the rules you've worked so hard to live by can feel like a step backwards, a weakness, but in actual fact it demonstrates immense bravery and strength.

It takes true grit and determination to maintain an illness such as orthorexia, and to follow a pattern of behaviour (in this case following the food rules) to the letter. I tell my clients that recovery is the time to use that energy and focus to genuinely improve their health – releasing themselves from the fear that drives their illness to instead experience true freedom and wellness.

Deciding to overcome an eating disorder is the first step on the road to recovery, but as I've already said the road is a long one. It's very important to surround yourself with emotional and psychological support, because the illness is the result of your mental health, rather than your physical health. You will need to be patient and determined in order to disentangle yourself from your negative sense of self-worth. Often things can feel like they are actually getting worse before they get better: once you pull the first thread, the unravelling can feel like complete chaos. This is why it's so important to make sure you have professional help to guide you through the process and a support network that will look after you into the future.

FINDING PROFESSIONAL HELP

We've already seen that there is a great deal of misinformation about, and a lack of clarity as to, who has a qualification to help you and who doesn't. It's very likely that if you have come to the realization that you or someone you love needs help, you won't want to ask around for a personal recommendation for a nutritionist, and especially for a mental health expert. I want to end the book with some advice and dos and don'ts on what to look for to find the right, qualified people to help you so that you can start your future in the right way.

Just as with treating other eating disorders, treating orthorexia is about healing the whole person – that is, it's not just about sorting out the diet or sorting out the mind, we need to do both. Sometimes, clients come to me when their mental health professional has identified that that particular sufferer needs nutritional intervention alongside their psychological therapy. In a high number of cases, though, I've found that an individual's first step is to self-refer to me, as they imagine they have a nutritional (rather than a psychological) problem. It might not be that they've realized they have an eating disorder (very often, it's not), but rather that some nutritional principle they're following isn't providing the expected physical results. They come to me in frustration, looking for me to tell them why their chosen nutritional path "isn't working". During my first assessment, if I suspect that a client has an eating disorder, I recommend that he or she seeks medical and psychological intervention to work alongside me. This means, first, a trip to their medical practitioner (that is, family doctor), who can then recommend a referral to a mental health professional and a dietitian (back to me, if possible).

In short, dealing with orthorexia requires a joined-up approach under general medical supervision to monitor overall physical health; a registered dietitian specializing in the field of eating disorders; and a mental health professional – a counsellor, psychotherapist or psychologist. You can start your journey with any one of these professionals – any one of them will help to find your way to the others, too.

Finding a nutritionist

If you have made it to this point in the book, then you've acknowledged that you or someone you know needs help. If I've convinced you now to ignore unsubstantiated claims on non-academic blogs and in unscientific news articles, you've taken another leap to getting better (or helping someone else to get better). So how do you actually choose a nutritionist or dietitian to help you?

First, please don't search for someone on the Internet – instead, talk to your medical practitioner and ask for a recommendation of a registered professional in your area. In some countries, the UK included, the job title "nutritionist" is not protected, so anyone from a personal trainer or an individual who has done a four-to-six week online diploma to someone who has spent years doing a degree can call him- or herself a nutritionist. In the US and Australia, there are more stringent controls over who can claim to be a nutritionist or dietitian, but even so things may vary from region to region or state to state – a recommendation from your medical health practitioner is the only way to be certain that you are talking to someone with the right nutritional qualifications and experience to help you.

To illustrate more clearly the minefield that this can be, and to ram home the point about how important it is that you get proper professional guidance on whom you talk to, the UK makes a very good example of how confusing it can be to find someone who is properly qualified to help. In the UK, nutritionists who have spent years studying usually have the letters RN, RNutr or UKVRN by their name – if you see these letters, you should be in good hands. Furthermore, the job title Dietitian is protected, and anyone carrying it has to have done the relevant degree or post-graduate degree university course in order to be accepted into the Health and Care Professions Council. This is the body that regulates all allied health practitioners, including (for example) psychologists, speech therapists, and physiotherapists. A qualified dietitian will usually show the letters RD (Registered Dietitian) after their name. However, the title nutritionist used without any letters and the title nutritional therapist are potentially unregulated. The table on pages 168–9 sets out the comparisons more clearly for the UK. In the USA, qualifications change depending on the state you're in, so it is even more important to consult your physician.

Once you've drawn up a shortlist of recommended registered nutritionists or dietitians in your area, find out about their areas of expertise before you commit. Not all clinicians will be experienced or qualified to work with eating disorders, which is a specialist area of nutrition that requires specific training that takes into account the behavioural and psychological aspects of these diseases. I've now worked in this field for more than 15 years, and training is ongoing and intense. I've attended conferences and completed short study modules, as well as also using both reflective practice and clinical supervision (by a clinical psychologist) to improve my knowledge. None of that is to say that you need to find someone with so much experience and training in the field – but some experience of eating disorders will ensure you get the best help available to you from the most qualified individuals.

It is also worth remembering that, although I've had some supervision from a clinical psychologist as part of my training, I am not a counsellor or psychologist.

My main role – and the role of any nutritionist or dietitian – is to address the issues surrounding food choice and to help each individual who comes to me with orthorexia understand the link between his or her emotions and the way he or she eats. It isn't to offer therapy or counselling itself – for this, every individual needs to see an expert in mental health (and eating disorders) alongside a nutritionist. My experience tells me that the combined approach gets the best results.

Finding a mental health expert

The best advice I can give you is to start with qualifications. Remember that orthorexia is an illness and therefore the professional help that you receive as part of your recovery needs to come with the appropriate regulatory gravitas. Many individuals who have an interest in psychology have set themselves up as life coaches and they are not qualified to provide the appropriate support in the case of a complex mental illness such as orthorexia.

In essence counsellors, psychotherapists and psychologists all do the same thing (using specific methods and practices to help you recover emotionally and behaviourally), but they take different approaches.

	Dietitian	
Is this a professionally recognized job title in the UK?	Yes	
What are the qualification requirements?	BSc in Dietetics or related science degree followed by a post-graduate qualification in Dietetics.	
Is the profession regulated by an independent body?	Yes All Dietitians have to be regulated by the Health and Care Professions Council (HCPC) in order to ensure that all their advice is evidence based and they practise while adhering to a strict code of conduct.	
Anything else I need to know?	Dietitians are the only qualified health professionals that assess, diagnose and treat dietary and nutritional problems at an individual and wider public health level. They work with both healthy and sick people in a variety of settings, from within a hospital or local medical practitioner to as specialists for sports teams.	

Nutritionist	Nutritional Therapist
No (anyone can call themselves a nutritionist), although a voluntary register (UKVRN) exists for Registered Nutritionists (with a degree qualification), whose work is audited (see below).	No
None, although in the UK courses that meet the strict standards of professional education in Nutrition are accredited by the Association for Nutrition (AFN). The UKVRN is run by the AFN.	None. Online courses are available and may vary in length from a few weeks to a year, and have varying standards of rigour.
No, although in the UK all nutritionists with a degree-related qualification are encouraged to register with the UKVRN (see top).	No Voluntary regulation is possible through the Complementary and Natural Healthcare Council (CNHC), but it is not compulsory. Also, this is self-regulated rather than independently regulated. Nutritional therapists in the UK are not eligible to register with either UKVRN or the HCPC.
Nutritionists may work in public health, health improvement, health policy, local and national government, in the private sector, Non-Government Organisations (NGOs) and in education and research.	Nutritional therapists work in private practice. They often provide advice on diet and lifestyle based on the principles of complementary (rather than conventional, scientific) medicine. They often offer advice on detoxification (including practices such as colonic irrigation) and the use of supplementary nutrients.

In general, psychotherapy encompasses all talking therapies, and the terms psychotherapist and counsellor are often used interchangeably. The key difference between psychotherapy and counselling is the length of time for treatment outcomes. Counselling usually refers to a shorter duration of therapy, focusing specifically on behavioural patterns. Psychotherapy is longer-term therapy, and aims to gain insight into the client's emotional problems and difficulties, helping him or her to become more self-aware of how their previous experiences affect their thoughts and behaviours.

In comparison, psychology is the study of the way people think, behave and interact. In order to obtain the title Psychologist, the practitioner will have completed a degree in Psychology. In order to then become a Counselling Psychologist, the practitioner would further need to obtain a doctorate in Counselling Psychology. A Counselling Psychologist can apply scientific understanding of the medical context of a mental health condition in ways that might not be available from counsellors or psychotherapists.

So what are the key differences between the different types of professional therapist and how do you relate this to choosing the right person to help you recover from orthorexia?

Counsellor

First, look for someone who is registered with one of
the following professional bodies in the UK or the USA
(as relevant), or the equivalent professional body in
your country:

- The British Association of Counselling and
  Psychotherapy (BACP)
- The UK Council for Psychotherapy (UKCP)
- The National Counselling Society (NCS)
- The American Psychological Association (APA)

A counsellor's aim will be to help you explore your
relationship with food, deciphering what it would
mean if you broke your food rules – in terms of how
that would make you feel, as well as the practical,
physical impact of doing so – and give you strategies
and techniques (such as turning your negative internal
narrative about certain foods into a positive one) to
help you cope with associated anxiety as you break
down the rules and learn to let them go.

For example, someone with orthorexia might become
agitated if he or she goes to the supermarket and
finds that their preferred brand of, say, yogurt is not
available. A counsellor gives strategies to manage this
anxiety and put it into perspective. In the joined-up

approach, at the same time, a dietitian will take the approach of educating and rationalizing, teaching that yogurt is yogurt and that one brand has the same effect on the body as another and will do just as well. This symbiotic relationship between practitioners and their client enables the sufferer to start to manage their emotions and re-establish reason in order that they can start to break down food rules and begin recovery.

Psychotherapist

First, look for someone who is registered with one of the following professional bodies in the UK or the USA, or the equivalent professional body in your country:

- The UK Council for Psychotherapy (UKCP)
- The American Psychological Association (APA)

A psychotherapist works at a slightly deeper level to a counsellor, trying to link present-day emotions and behaviours with past experiences, in order to identify how those past experiences can have manifested in orthorexia. Improving self-awareness in this way, and understanding how things that happen to us have a ripple effect that can influence other aspects of our lives, helps to improve self-compassion. This, in turn, enables the sufferer to improve their ability to manage their negative emotions, understanding where they come from and why he or she has them, and so treating them and responding to them appropriately.

Remember that in orthorexia the aim is to purify the body, which the sufferer believes he or she can achieve through dietary control. A psychotherapist will explore the notion of purity and try to understand why his or her client feels that the body needs cleansing in the first place. The trigger might be something far back in time – perhaps an episode of bullying, a difficult relationship with a parent or sibling, or a bereavement or other loss that has resulted in deep-rooted feelings of lack of self worth – of not feeling deserving of love or care. A psychotherapist helps his or her client to understand that the desire to be pure is linked to the internal psychological struggle. In effect, the struggle is not really triggered by or even related to food or eating, but to negative emotions about the sufferer him- or herself. Step by step, a psychotherapist helps individuals to change how they feel about themselves, providing the tools to reset their self-compassion.

Working alongside a psychotherapist, the dietitian helps orthorexia sufferers to understand how they transfer their negative emotions onto food choice. So, for example, during recovery, a dietitian will encourage sufferers to try foods that they have placed on their own banned list. The psychotherapy route explores how this positive step – eating something that is good for you, but has been somehow demonized through illness – can result in feelings of guilt and embarrassment. Not because the food itself is "bad", but because at this point in recovery the sufferer realizes that eating that food is a positive step, but they don't feel worthy of taking that step, of doing something good for themselves. Both dietitian and psychotherapist help to provide rational voices to help individuals understand that they deserve and need to take forward steps, to break their food rules in order to save their health.

Psychologist

First, look for someone with the following qualifications, or the equivalent in your country, and who is registered with the following professional bodies (again, or equivalent):

- The psychologist should have a British Psychology Society (BPS) accredited degree, specialist work experience and then a further BPS accredited post-graduate qualification in eating disorders; he or she should be regulated by the Health and Care Professions Council in the UK.

- He or she should be regulated by the American Board of Professional Psychology in the USA.

Psychologists use a combination of both counselling and psychotherapy. They are also able to prescribe medication for low mood and anxiety based on a medical and psychological assessment – bearing in mind that, in severe cases, orthorexic individuals will suffer not only with high levels of anxiety, but also with depression stemming from feelings of being trapped in their own food rules. In these cases, a psychologist can step in and prescribe medication that can just lift anxiety temporarily so that the individual can feel more rational and so engage in counselling more effectively.

There is no set rule relating to, or particular sequence for, whom you should choose to work with. Whether you end up with a counsellor, psychotherapist or psychologist may come down to availability and expertise in your area, as not all therapists in all forms will have expertise in treating eating disorders. Most importantly, you need to be at complete ease with your practitioner and you need to be able to form a connection, rapport and bond.

Developing trust

While how you feel about your mental health practitioner may not be obvious after your first meeting, within a few sessions you should know whether or not you are building a rapport and are starting to feel safe in their company. This on-going clinical relationship is critical to your recovery, so it is important that you do feel able to be completely open and honest. And, don't be afraid to change therapists if something isn't working. Often individuals worry about having to start all over again, or somehow offending the therapist they are working with – your recovery from orthorexia is the most important thing. A good clinician will respect you for putting your recovery first.

MAINTAINING YOUR RECOVERY

Once you have come to the end of the clinical road of recovery – the point at which your nutritionist and therapist think you are well enough to work on your own, it's so important that you practise self-help that enables you to stay on track long into the future. Some of the following suggestions will give you the space you may need to reflect on the work you have done with your dietitian and therapist; others will help you continue to change your negative narrative into a positive one that reinforces your sense of self-worth every day.

Give yourself time to appreciate

My friend, author Emma Woolf, in her book *Positively Primal*, talks about the importance and art of appreciation. She recommends trying to appreciate three things a day. This could be the first cup of steaming coffee, the view from your bedroom window or that moment when you have finished work or tidying up and you just sit down finally and are able to switch off.

Orthorexia is a complicated illness closely linked with self-esteem and self-worth issues and an orthorexic finds it difficult to let him- or herself off the hook; there's no downtime from the pressure of remaining pure, the whip is constantly cracking and the pursuit of perfection removes all pleasure from life. Taking time to stop, appreciate and be grateful for even the simplest things can help to shift that mindset, little by little restoring a sense of pleasure in simplicity.

Be mindful of the latest eating fads

When you are on the road to recovery from orthorexia, it is important to remember that what is the "big thing" in terms of eating-fad today is likely to be replaced with something new – even something totally contradictory – tomorrow. Nothing in the world of pseudo-nutrition ever stands still. Why? Because no fad or dietary regime holds the answer to emotional and physical perfection – that (as we've said) comes from within. This point is as important for someone in the grip of orthorexia as it is for those who are at the start of their road to recovery and those who are nearing the end of their journey or who have returned to wellness for a while. Always be on the lookout for anything that might draw you back in, and keep up the positive self-talk: you *are* good enough.

CASE STUDY

POWER IS WITHIN

I was talking to a client of mine the other day. She has been well for some time and has fully appreciated that her orthorexia had kept her a prisoner. She is now living life rather than just surviving. However, she has recently found herself becoming increasingly more critical of her eating. She has noticed feelings of guilt and anxiety related to consuming foods she had once deemed "unpure". Her work with her psychiatrist and with me had empowered her enough to notice where her mind was taking her. She asked herself why, and she concluded that a recent extended visit to her family (whom she loves to see) had triggered old feelings of not being good enough. She had almost returned to her default position – punishing herself through food choice – but her self-awareness made her realize that she had it in her power to stop her relapse.

This story illustrates how easy it is to resort to old patterns of thinking and behaving – so, whether it's a deep-rooted insecurity or a new diet fad that seems appealing, be alert.

Switch off social media

Okay, I accept that in this day and age, social media is a way to stay connected to friends near and far, so if you can't switch off from social media completely, disconnect yourself from any groups that do not serve you (dieting blogs, celebrity blogs, exercise sites and so on) and make social media just that – a form of socializing with those you love who perhaps you don't see very often. Try to give yourself a digital detox every now and then – cold turkey on the digital social platforms. Even just a few hours a week, or a whole weekend will help you realize that there is much more to life than what's happening on your screen. If you can remove yourself from it altogether, so much the better. Many of my clients have spoken about the huge relief they have felt when they deleted their Facebook, Instagram, Twitter and Snapchat accounts – they no longer felt the pressure to conform to ideals that weren't real for them.

Do yoga

Although it's not essential for maintaining your recovery, yoga is a wonderful way to fill time in a positive physical and mental way. If sufferers have also become obsessive about exercise, yoga provides physical exertion, but also time to reflect in a form of moving meditation. By focusing on breathing and moving through postures, you should find that you create a little space and time for you to stop and focus on yourself.

Be kind to yourself

Up until the point you established your recovery, you were expending huge amounts of your attention, time and energy on eating and living in a particular way – a way that wasn't healthy for you. Since then, you redirected that energy into your recovery. Now you need to channel that energy into learning to be self-compassionate *at all times*, reminding yourself that no-one is perfect and nothing you eat, drink or wear is going to make you so.

Focus on surrounding yourself with the people who make you feel good about yourself, feed off their positivity but remember that the positivity itself comes from within you. Let yourself off the hook. If you are tired, then rest. If you are sad, then cry. If you are lonely, then reach out to a friend. If you are hungry, think about what you really want to eat – if it is chocolate, then allow yourself to have it. Enjoy it; appreciate every mouthful and tell yourself how delicious it is. Keep praising yourself for following your instincts and being true to yourself.

RAISING AWARENESS: A NEED

Finally, I want to look at what the medical profession and clinical researchers are doing, and need to do, in order to turn the tide on this dangerous eating disorder.

At the time of writing, one of the most recent (pre-published online at the end of March 2017) studies concludes that compared with other eating disorders, such as anorexia and bulimia, orthorexia is not yet treated seriously among the general public – but then how can it be when there's so little information about it? The research concluded that it's seen as a lifestyle choice, rather than a mental disorder – people choose to eat healthily, rather than people find themselves victim of a compulsive need to punish themselves through diet restriction. The dangers of orthorexia are very real, though – especially if it isn't yet properly perceived as a disorder among those who might be most vulnerable. And that's what the future needs to change.

It is highly possible that orthorexia has existed for many years, but, if we extrapolate modern attitudes, it's likely that it has continually been dismissed as lifestyle choice. Think back through your own life and relationships: you may have experienced a friend who has become obsessive about certain dietary rules, but you just accepted these as something he or she wanted as part of his or her lifestyle. Even if that friend withdrew from life (perhaps you saw him or her less than you used to), you might have passed that off as the transience of friendship – after all, life takes us in different directions all the time. If we don't know about something, if there's no awareness of a potential problem, we aren't alert to the signs it is there. (If, on the other hand, the same friend had been starving him- or herself, alarm bells may have gone off; you may have asked yourself, could this person be suffering from an eating disorder? Because you already know about and understand the basic principles and signs of, for example, anorexia.)

As I mentioned at the start of this book, deciphering who is suffering is one of the most difficult aspects of orthorexia, as the illness can so easily be hidden under the guise of healthy eating. Who can really contradict someone if they are basing the majority of their nutritional intake on the consumption of supposedly healthy fruit and vegetables?

Clinical research

As I've already said, clinically speaking orthorexia is a fairly new phenomenon, so research into the field is still scarce. If you put a search for orthorexia into PubMed (the website that catalogues medical research papers and findings), only 65 journal articles come up, with the majority of research having been conducted in only the last few years. But, things are changing – we are raising awareness and increasingly researchers are realizing that we need more investigations into this important, growing area of health.

That said, orthorexia is currently receiving a huge amount of interest, resulting in new areas of research looking at the epidemiology, potential risk factors, treatment options, and outcomes.

THE ORTHOREXIA TEST – FINDING A DIAGNOSTIC TOOL

There is still much controversy as to whether or not it is possible to have a diagnostic tool (a test, for want of a better term) for orthorexia. While Dr. Steven Bratman (see page 7) initially proposed a ten-item rating scale by which to measure orthorexia, an alternative is now in circulation, known as ORTO-15. I have chosen not to reproduce the test in the book because it is the subject of great debate. It asks 15 questions based on interpreting patterns of behaviour relating to food. Some questions relate to preoccupation with calories, evaluation of the "healthiness" of food, feelings and thoughts about food, and how we relate food to our appearance or sense of well-being. Others ask if we're prepared to spend money on perceived healthy foods, or how food relates to our sociability. Each question is scored 1 to 4 depending upon whether it relates to you always, often, sometimes or never. Scores are totted up and then an analysis of orthorexia, orthorexic tendencies or healthy attitudes to food ensues. The problem is that demographics, mood, disposable income and so many other transient factors can influence the outcome. In addition, many of the questions aren't specific to orthorexia and so aren't pinpointed enough to provide confident diagnosis.

It's now widely accepted that we need something better. With the rise in incidence and increased awareness that orthorexia exists, producing a diagnostic tool that clinicians can use universally is high on the agenda. At the time of writing, Dr. Bratman and his colleague Thom Dunn have recently launched an initiative to collect data that might enable them to improve on the ORTO-15, perhaps paring it down rather than expanding it, to give a more precise diagnostic tool. Only once we can more accurately diagnose orthorexia as a medical condition can we hope to have it officially recognized as an eating disorder in the *DSM*-5 (see box, page 9).

Tackling the social media problem

I am aware that it is easy to blame social media for increasing the risks of eating disorders such as orthorexia. However, since I began treating sufferers of this condition, it has become my belief that social media, and those who post healthy, perfect images of themselves alongside diet advice unfounded in any nutritional expertise, have a lot to answer for. Overall, statistics indicate that less than 1 per cent of the population suffers from orthorexia (remembering, though, that this statistic could be skewed by the difficulties in recognizing and diagnosing the condition). However, a research paper published in March 2017 looked specifically for a link between susceptibility to orthorexia or orthorexic mindsets and the use of Instagram. In the cohort of more than 600 participants, the researchers found that almost half the people (49 per cent) who took part in an online survey showed attitudes and behaviours characteristic of orthorexia. When less than 1 per cent of the population in general shows these tendencies, the influence of social media seems blatantly clear.

As a registered dietitian and regulated nutritional practitioner, I am passionate about educating people on the true value of good, balanced nutrition. In the future I want anyone looking for dietary advice to go to credible, scientific sources, to seek out registered experts rather than turning to pseudo-nutritionists who, wishing only to tell their good-luck story, inadvertently mislead and misrepresent.

Credible scientific studies look at large population groups and test specific nutritional theories. This is how dietitians and registered nutritionists know what advice to give to their clients. It's not even just a case of looking at published studies and drawing your own conclusions (although, this is better than reading unqualified and unsubstantiated dietary information) – after all, not all research is equivalent. To be really safe, you need to meet with or talk to someone who has the right qualifications to be able to critically appraise a paper and understand its evidence in light of other pieces of scientific evidence already in circulation.

Knowing whom to trust

Interestingly, the backlash against "clean eating" seems to have started with many of the original advocates of this lifestyle distancing themselves from their own claims. It doesn't undo the damage that's been done, of course, but it does start to redress the balance for the future. My hope is that those people who have trusted bloggers and Instagrammers in the past will now realize that not all the diet and lifestyle advice they read was worth adopting; and that not all the images they saw were in fact "real" (see pages 32–5).

Glamourized images and messages are hard to reverse – but not impossible. The true experts just need to shout louder. There does seem to be a lot of good work coming through from professional nutritionists and dietitians hoping to help the public re-educate themselves about what a healthy diet actually means. Blogs, articles and books by the likes of Bee Wilson, the Angry Chef (aka Anthony Warner), Fight the Fads, and the Rooted project are starting to gather good followings as word spreads that all that glisters is not gold. They aren't quite matching the numbers of followers you see on celebrity blogs and Instagram accounts, but things are getting there. We just need to keep raising awareness.

The single, most important message I want to get across is: be wary of where you get your information. Remember that anyone can call themselves a nutritionist, but it is only those with a Dietetic or Nutrition first degree or masters degree who are regulated and registered to provide you with information on diet and nutrition that you know you can trust. My biggest hope for the future is that individuals – and particularly teenagers – start to understand that social media is just a snapshot of a moment in time; it is not reality and no one should use it or its click-counters as a barometer of reliability.

Of course, though, anyone who is susceptible to orthorexia is more likely to trust an ill-founded source of information than something that has been well researched but that doesn't validate their own behaviours. Remember, however, that being good at marketing an idea or theory you have, or a practice that works for you, does not make you an expert in that field. Registered nutritionists and dietitians are academic experts – that might not sound very glamorous, but then glamour is rarely all it's cracked up to be.

A FINAL WORD

In 2016 I was invited as a professional and qualified clinical and sports dietitian to sit on a panel at the Cheltenham Literature Festival. The aim was for me to offer a scientific and academic perspective on the notion of clean eating. The other panellists were Bee Wilson, a highly respected food historian and writer, and a well-known and successful food blogger, who had experienced a turnaround in her health that she attributed to changes in her diet.

It was an interesting and heated debate, and I was surprised at how unwilling members of the audience were to heed scientific over circumstantial evidence. It showed me unequivocally that we are all searching for a miracle cure and we want it at all costs and against all reason. When someone offers that cure – regardless of whether or not he or she has any evidence for it other than personal experience – we want to believe. And we don't like it when someone else tells us that science proves otherwise.

The term "clean eating" commonly appears on blogs and in books as a synonym for "healthy eating". For me, then, clean eating is a dangerous term. It implies that eating any other way is somehow unclean. As I've already said, I define healthy eating as unrestrained eating – everything in moderation. I realize that's not sexy or innovative, and I realize it's probably the last thing that anyone searching for a nutritional miracle really wants to hear. But, sometimes it's the obvious, safe path that leads us to where we want to go.

I don't think food and fitness regimes cause eating disorders – an eating disorder is a very complicated multifactorial mental illness. However, those with orthorexia follow food rules, and "clean eating" – whether that manifests as gluten-free, dairy-free or sugar-free, or anything else – provides rules. Pretty much every single eating disorder individual I have worked with – young, old, male, female, athlete, non-athlete – talks about the rules. And when those who make up the rules are young, beautiful, successful and skinny, the incentive to follow them to reach perfection is too tempting to resist.

I stand by my word that being healthy is not just about food; it is also a mindset. I hope that if you are a sufferer or someone who cares about a sufferer, you have learned in this book that life doesn't need to be lived by food rules, and that a shift in thinking, a releasing of self-induced pressure and unrealistic expectation can have a dramatically positive effect on health and well-being – in a way that old rules can't. In addition, when we remove the pleasure of eating and replace it with fear and anxiety, we all have cause for concern.

I try to teach my daughters and my clients that the most powerful routes to success and well-being are self-acceptance and self-worth. These don't come from eating a certain way or following a certain practice: self-esteem comes from accepting that you are good enough just the way you are.

RESOURCES

· ·

There is only so much a book can ever do – recovery from any illness, but especially an illness with psychological effects, is individual and unique to each sufferer. If you think you or someone you know is suffering from orthorexia, get in touch with any of the following organizations, who will be able to offer you advice about how to receive the best treatment and begin your path to recovery.

IN THE UK

· ·

Anorexia and Bulimia Care (ABC)

www.anorexiabulimiacare.org.uk
A national eating disorder charity that has a full-time helpline for anyone who is struggling, or caring for someone, with any form of eating disorder. The charity also provides training and education to schools,

universities, the workplace, and NHS trusts. Every November they have an action month during which ABC campaigns for better resources available to help understand and combat eating disorders. The action month has been launched at the Houses of Parliament for the last four years.

BEAT

www.b-eat.co.uk/support-services
A national eating disorder charity that offers helpline services most evenings of the week. The charity also provides education and support and continues to raise awareness of eating disorders.

Student Minds

www.studentminds.org.uk
The UK's student mental health charity offers support groups within university settings covering a range of mental-health issues, including eating disorders.

Finding professional help

As I have said in the book, it is best that you talk to your medical practitioner for a recommendation of a registered, qualified counsellor, psychologist, psychotherapist or dietitian in your area. If you'd like to check the list you're given by your surgery, you can use the following links, which are a reliable directory of qualified mental and nutritional health providers in the UK.

Finding a dietitian

www.bda.uk.com/improvinghealth/yourhealth/finddietitian

Finding a registered nutritionist

www.associationfornutrition.org

Finding a counsellor

www.counselling-directory.org.uk

Finding a psychologist

www.bps.org.uk/psychology-public/find-psychologist/find-psychologist

Finding a psychotherapist

www.psychotherapy.org.uk

IN THE US

Healthcare provision and treatment in the USA varies enormously, depending on the state, and regulations are changing all the time. If you are concerned about yourself or someone you know, talk to your physician, and speak to agencies that are based in your location. The following resources are a springboard to those services.

National Eating Disorders Association (NEDA)

www.nationaleatingdisorders.org
NEDA supports individuals and families affected by eating disorders, and is the leading non-profit in this area. Their helpline is a useful first stop for anyone worried about an eating disorder.

Alliance for Eating Disorders Awareness (The Alliance)

www.allianceforeatingdisorders.com
This agency aims to connect people seeking help for eating disorders with resources and information to assist them in their recovery. They offer workshops and presentations, free support groups for those struggling and for their loved ones, advocacy for eating disorders and mental health legislation, national toll-free phone help line, and referrals, support and mentoring services.

Eating Disorder HOPE

www.eatingdisorderhope.com
This umbrella organization offers hope, information and resources to people with various eating disorders,

their family members, and treatment providers. They can help refer you to eating disorder organizations and services in your state.

ACKNOWLEDGEMENTS

This book has been a real labour of love. It is a book that I have wanted to write for such a long time and I am so grateful to Watkins Media and Nourish Books for supporting and backing me on this project. To Bee Wilson for providing me with a Foreword, thank you so much (check out Bee's brilliant book – *This is Not a Diet Book* – which explores why diets and fads don't work). There is one person whom I have to thank above all others when it comes to this book, and that is my brilliant editor Judy Barratt. Without your patience and guidance, I'm not sure there would have been a book, so thank you for just being wonderful.

A huge thank you to my beautiful daughters, Maya and Ella, who keep me grounded and who remind me at regular intervals, while I'm writing, to breathe and to take our spaniel Bailey out for a long walk or a run.

Thank you to my parents and sister for doing what families do best.

A huge thank you to my amazing friends who have supported me through this journey, reminding me of the importance and relevance of, and need for, such a book, especially at the times when I've ground to a complete halt. There are a few of you who cannot go unnamed: so thank you to Holly, Sarah, Pete, PM, Dom, Lizzie, Dee, Claire, Eloise, Amy, Ewen, Nick, Philippa and Alison.

One final thank you to the Chief Executive of ABC charity, Jane Smith, for her tireless work for the charity and for leading such a brilliant team of individuals, who help people suffering from eating disorders every single day.

INDEX

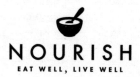

NOURISH
EAT WELL, LIVE WELL

Here at Nourish we're all about wellbeing through food and drink –
irresistible dishes with a serious good-for-you factor. If you want to eat and
drink delicious things that set you up for the day, suit any special diets,
keep you healthy and make the most of the ingredients you have, we've
got some great ideas to share with you. Come over to our blog for
wholesome recipes and fresh inspiration – nourishbooks.com

About the Author

Renee McGregor BSc(Hons) PGDip(Diet) RD PgCert (Sportsnutr) SENr is a Performance and Clinical Dietitan, accredited by the Health Professions Council and Sports Exercise and Nutrition register (SENr). With years of experience and expertise in sports nutrition, she advises athletes at amateur, professional and Olympic level. In 2016 she attended the Paralympic Games in Rio where she was supporting wheelchair basketball and wheelchair fencing athletes, and she is looking forward to being involved in the Tokyo cycle in 2020.

Renee's clinical area of expertise lies in eating disorders and she provides support and advice to all, with a crossover into her sports nutrition. She is the Clinical Nutrition Lead at ABC, the Anorexia and Bulimia Charity in the UK. She has presented at conferences, been a panelist on the "Clean Eating Debate" at the Cheltenham Literature Festival, spoken on radio and podcasts, and written guest blogs and articles for national publications. Renee is also the author of *Training Food*, *Fast Fuel: Food for Triathalon Success* and *Fast Fuel: Food for Running Success* for Nourish.